Accountability in Nursing and Midwifery

Second edition

Edited by

Stephen Tilley
BA, RMN, PhD

Senior Lecturer, Nursing Studies
University of Edinburgh
Edinburgh

and

Roger Watson
BSc PhD RGN CBiol FIBiol ILTM FRSA

Professor of Nursing
School of Nursing, Social Work and Applied Health Studies
University of Hull
Hull

Blackwell
Science

NLGIB GSTK (EKGOF)

Editorial offices:
Blackwell Science Ltd, 9600 Garsington Road, Oxford OX4 2DQ, UK
    Tel: +44 (0) 1865 776868
Blackwell Publishing Inc., 350 Main Street, Malden, MA 02148-5020, USA
    Tel: +1 781 388 8250
Blackwell Science Asia Pty Ltd, 550 Swanston Street, Carlton, Victoria 3053, Australia
    Tel: +61 (0)3 8359 1011

First edition published by Chapman & Hall 1995
Second edition published by Blackwell Science Ltd 2004
Reprinted 2005

Library of Congress Cataloging-in-Publication Data

Accountability in nursing and midwifery / edited by Stephen Tilley and
Roger Watson.—2nd ed.
        p. ; cm.
Rev. ed. of: Accountability in nursing practice / edited by Roger
Watson. London : Chapman & Hall, 1995.
Includes bibliographical references and index.
        ISBN 0-632-06469-2 (pbk. : alk. paper)
    1. Nursing—Standards—Great Britain. 2. Midwifery—Standards—Great
Britain. 3. Responsibility. 4. Clinical competence.
        [DNLM: 1. Midwifery—standards. 2. Nursing—standards. 3. Nursing
Care—standards. 4. Quality Assurance, Health Care. WY 16 A172 2004]
I. Tilley, Stephen. II. Watson, Roger, 1955– III. Accountability in
nursing practice.

        RT85.5.A25 2004
        610.73'06'9—dc22

                                                2003020922

ISBN-10: 0-632-06469-2
ISBN-13: 978-0632-06469-4

A catalogue record for this title is available from the British Library

Set in 10.5/12.5pt Sabon
by Graphicraft Limited, Hong Kong
Printed and bound by Replika Press Pvt. Ltd, India

For further information on Blackwell Publishing, visit our website:
www.blackwellnursing.com

Contents

Contributors

Sarah Baggaley
BSc SRN SCM HV
Lecturer, Nursing Studies, University of Edinburgh

Alison Bryans
BA MSc RGN HV RNT
Research Fellow/Lecturer, Department of Nursing and Community
Health, Glasgow Caledonian University

Gosia M. Brykczyñska
BA BSc PhD RGN/RGCN RNT Cev
Consultant to International Department of RCN, Freelance Lecturer,
London

Bob Gates
MSc BEd(Hons) Dip Nurs (Lond) RNMH RMN RNT Cert Ed
Head of Learning Disabilities, Thames Valley University, Berkshire

Tracey Heath
RGN BSc(Hons) MSc
Lecturer/Senior Nurse, Evidence-Based Practice, School of Nursing, Social
Work and Applied Health Studies, The University of Hull

Tony Hostick
RMN MSc MIQA
Head of Research and Effectiveness, Hull & East Riding Community
Health NHS Trust, Honorary Fellow, School of Nursing, Social Work and
Applied Health Studies, University of Hull

Kerry Jacobs
PhD CA(Nr)
Professor of Accounting, La Trobe University, Melbourne. Formerly
Senior Lecturer, School of Management, University of Edinburgh

Stephen Knight
MPhil BPhil RN RNT RCNT
Divisional Nurse, Medical Division, Hull & East Yorkshire Hospitals
NHS Trust, Hull Royal Infirmary

Rosemary Mander
MSc PhD RGM SCM MTD
Reader, Nursing Studies, University of Edinburgh

Susan McGann
BA (Hons)
Archivist, Royal College of Nursing, Edinburgh

Linda C. Pollock
BSc RGN DIM Diploma in Clinical Nursing RMN PhD MBA
Nursing Director, Lothian Primary Care Trust, Astley Ainslie Hospital,
Edinburgh

Alison Tierney
BSc PhD RN FRCN CBE
Professor, Department of Clinical Nursing, University of Adelaide, South
Australia; Formerly Professor of Nursing Research, University of Edinburgh

Stephen Tilley
BA PhD RMN JBCNS 650
Senior Lecturer, Nursing Studies, University of Edinburgh, Edinburgh

John Tingle
BA Law Hons Cert Ed (Dist) MEd Barrister
Reader in Health Law, Nottingham Law School, Nottingham Trent
University

Jane Wray
RGN BA(Hons) HETC Dip Aromatherapy (IIHHT) MPhil
Research Associate, The East Yorkshire Disability Institute, University of Hull

Michael Wolverson
RNMH BA(Hons) MSc
Lecturer, Department of Health Studies, University of York

Roger Watson
BSc PhD RGN CBiol FIBiol ILTM FRSA
Professor of Nursing, School of Nursing, Social Work and Applied Health
Studies, University of Hull

Preface

Roger Watson

The first edition of this book (Watson, 1995) was a landmark in the sense that it was the first textbook to deal exclusively with the issue of accountability in nursing. The present edition has similarities to and differences from the first edition. The similarities are necessary in order to provide continuity and are represented by some of the original authors being involved. The differences are essential and are represented by some additional authors and also by developments in some of the original chapters.

The introduction to the first edition dwelt on the nature of accountability and its application to nursing. The essential features were teased out and the second editor reckoned that accountability was an essential feature of professionalism in a world where the question of whether nursing practice is professional was still in doubt. The original arguments will not be rehearsed here as they are analysed fully in one of the chapters in this edition. Furthermore, the world of healthcare has moved on, such that the professional nature of nursing is hardly brought into question.

However, the world in which nursing and midwifery now have to operate is quite different and a major new feature is clinical governance. It was felt by editors, publishers and reviewers of the original proposal alike that any consideration of accountability in nursing and midwifery which did not include clinical governance would be incomplete. In order to address this, therefore, the present volume includes contributions from practice which examine the issue of clinical governance from a number of perspectives and also chapters in which the link between accountability and clinical governance is examined.

Two of the major issues of the introduction to the first edition were to whom nurses were accountable and how they dealt with multiple forms of accountability. Accountability, at the time of the first edition, was something which nurses claimed, although not universally. Nurses also had conflicting ideas of who they were accountable to and this ranged from being accountable to patients to being accountable to their employers, with accountability to their professional body, the United Kingdom Central Council for Nursing, Midwifery and Health Visiting, included somewhere in the spectrum.

The advent of clinical governance has, on the one hand, brought account-ability into clearer focus and, on the other hand, changed the nature of account-ability in nursing. Clinical governance provides a framework, essentially lacking in previous years, within which nurses and other healthcare professionals must work. The nature of accountability is highly specified in guidelines for practice and protocols for patient care. On the other hand, the notion of accountability based on education and training, which defined nursing as a profession, may have been eroded as there is less scope for individuals to act accountably in a given set of circumstances. Rather, the circumstances in which nurses and midwives are expected to work and how they are expected to work in terms of outcomes are more specific.

In the present volume, arguments from both sides of the debate about whether clinical governance, and other associated developments, are a good thing for nursing and whether or not they enhance professional accountability will be presented. Clinical governance will not go away and there are many legitimate reasons for its inception. However, readers are asked to consider whether or not this is a positive development for them as nurses and mid-wives and whether or not the many other changes we are witnessing to nurse education and career development are heading in the right direction.

In common with the production of the first edition, many authors – espe-cially those new to this edition – were worried that they would merely repeat the material of other authors. This, of course, is predicated upon the premise that repetition is, of itself, wrong. Naturally, there is some repeti-tion. Certainly, the authors all draw upon a similar set of sources but this is to be expected. They are all looking at the same phenomena from differ-ent perspectives. On the other hand, in common with the first edition, there is remarkably little repetition. Each author or set of authors has taken a unique line on accountability and clinical governance. This was due to the selection of topics for the second edition, the unique perspectives of the authors and also to the fact that both accountability and clinical governance are open to interpretation. Definitions of accountability and clinical governance exist but it is how these impact upon different areas of practice and different levels of responsibility in healthcare that provides the perspectives. The Introduction takes each chapter in turn and provides an editor's perspective on each. However, these are not summaries and each chapter is worthy of study in its own right.

Chapter 1
Introduction

Roger Watson & Stephen Tilley

Historical perspective

Susan McGann traces the development of nursing as an accountable profession. Achieving professional status was a struggle for nurses, and modern developments can be traced to 1919 and the passing of the Nurses' Registration Act. The involvement of nurses in World War I played a significant part in bringing this Act to the statute books and a key person in this was Mrs Bedford Fenwick, supported by her physician husband. The registration of nurses had been opposed by Florence Nightingale, who was more concerned with the character of nurses than with their entry on a register. However, Florence Nightingale died before World War I and one of her supporters in the fight against registration died in 1919 – perhaps this was significant. The historical and political perspective on the development of professional nursing offered by McGann, taking us up to 1919 and establishing the historical basis for claims of accountability linked to professional registration, continues to inform the ongoing debate about accountability in nursing.

An accountant looks at nursing

Kerry Jacobs brings a welcome critical perspective in his chapter. Jacobs essentially considers the definition and scope of accountability and how this applies to nursing. Much of the debate about accountability in nursing stems from Lewis & Batey's (and Batey & Lewis') seminal papers, which are usually referred to without question or criticism. Jacobs is forthright in his assertion that Lewis & Batey were wrong about accountability and, therefore, wrong about the implications for nursing. For those of us who have taken Lewis & Batey, if not as the starting point for the debate about accountability in nursing then certainly as a pivotal point, this has serious implications. Essentially our arguments may be flawed. Jacobs considers the assertion that accountability is the hallmark of professionalism (Watson, 1995 introduction) to be, at the very least, incomplete.

A profession such as nursing, which at one point in its history was striving to be considered accountable and therefore a profession, was only

seeing one side of the accountability coin. In fact, such a struggle for accountability may have been naive to the extent that accountability is imposed rather
than self-claimed, and nursing, and other healthcare professions, including
medicine, have now imposed accountability in large measure. While nursing was striving for and trying to define its accountability, it may have played
into the hands of those who sought to impose greater levels of accountability without any regard for professional development. Jacobs draws attention
to dangers stemming from a structural perspective on accountabilty which
emphasises 'domination and control', and instead endorses the value of a
'discourse of individual accountability in nursing'.

Accountability and clinical governance

Clinical governance has been a relatively recent addition to the guidelines
for working with patients in the NHS. The second editor examines the relationship between accountability in nursing and midwifery and clinical governance. If accountability is still the hallmark of a profession, as he asserts,
then the question arises as to whether or not clinical governance enhances
that professionalism through its effect on accountability. There is plenty of
opinion from outside nursing and midwifery – principally from medicine –
about the damaging effects of clinical governance, and all of its components,
on the work of doctors. Much of this is directly applicable to nursing and
is perhaps even more relevant here as clinical governance appears to strike
at the heart of the relationship between the professional and the patient and
nursing is, essentially, all about that relationship.

The Reith lectures of 2002, in which the issue of trust was examined, are
drawn upon to support the argument that clinical governance is just another
aspect of how the trust between the public and professionals is being eroded.
We seem to have entered a period where risk is not an option and every interaction between professionals and the public must be prescribed in scope and
recorded in detail. The conclusion of this chapter is that clinical governance,
a manifestation of lack of trust, is not conducive to accountability.

Accountability and the law

The main change to take place in the wake of clinical governance, according
to Tingle, is that the patient has been put at the centre of government policy in relation to the NHS. This can be seen in the relevant legislation and
establishment of bodies such as the Commission for Health Improvement
(CHI) and the National Patient Safety Agency (NPSA). Clearly, legal
accountability is one particular type of accountability but nurses need to be
aware of the ways in which they may be accountable to the law and the ways
in which their work may open up their employers to legal proceedings
through their vicarious liability. The purpose of the law is not just to
punish but also to provide deterrence and to provide compensation when

things go wrong. Nurses are accountable in a great many ways and many penalties can be imposed outside the law. However, the harshest penalties rest with the law and it is the wise nurse or midwife who has, at least, a working knowledge of their legal liability.

The problem of multiple accountability is raised by Tingle and the example of poor staffing levels is used to illustrate this: nurses are accountable to their employer but also to the Nursing and Midwifery Council for the standards of care they deliver. In the case where something goes wrong then the law has a hard job to decide an outcome. As Tingle argues, the law cannot be seen to sanction poor standards of care but must also offer reasonable protection to those working under difficult circumstances.

A policy perspective

Tracey Heath provides an overview of the policies relevant to accountability and clinical governance. An important shift has been made from implicit to explicit accountability and this is now visible in what Heath describes as the 'bold type' of Government policy. In many ways, it is remarkable to look back at landmarks in NHS management, such as the Griffiths Report in the early 1980s, which saw the introduction of general management in the NHS, and the reforms of the late 1980s which introduced the purchaser-provider split into the NHS in an effort to increase efficiency and patient care. Those days seem long gone but the web of legislation around the NHS remains. According to Heath, who takes a generally positive view of clinical governance, the reforms of the post-1997 Labour Government were building on previous Conservative legislation. However, the purchaser-provider concept and market forces have been replaced by a range of new bodies each purporting to oversee accountability in the NHS within the framework of clinical governance.

An NHS trust perspective

Stephen Knight and Tony Hostick provide a view of clinical governance from within two NHS trusts: one acute and one community trust respectively. Accountability, within a clinical governance framework, is traced from the individual level through the trust level and a stepped approach to decision making is presented as one way of approaching the demands of clinical governance. Delivery of quality lies at the heart of clinical governance and NHS chief executives are responsible for delivering quality care and, therefore, are also responsible for the quality of professional decision making within their domains of responsibility. In addition to the above, clinical governance also implies user involvement and continuing professional development and these have implications for individuals and NHS trusts.

Clinical governance is very visible within NHS trusts through the implementation of the seven technical components of clinical governance, listed by Knight & Hostick, and these require a committee structure reporting to the NHS trust board and, ultimately, to the Department of Health through the Strategic Health Authorities, in England. The 'top-down' view of NHS trusts is the extent to which they can demonstrate evidence-based decision making built on the aggregate of clinical governance outcomes at all levels in the trust and across the range of the seven technical components. However, Knight & Hostick argue that the real responsibility of NHS trusts is to create the right environment for staff to be clinically effective through the provision of policies and training.

Professional self-regulation, which may be under threat in the era of clinical governance, as argued elsewhere in this book, through the application of the 'tick box' mentality and the erosion of trust in professionals, is clearly part of clinical governance through the aim of regulation, which is to protect the public. Knight & Hostick take a fairly neutral view of clinical governance and this is perhaps indicative of the fact that they are obliged to implement it without the luxury of viewing it from an academic perspective. As such, their contribution is very valuable.

A manager speaks

Linda Pollock provides an enthusiastic view of clinical governance from the perspective of a nursing director in the NHS in Scotland. The Scottish situation is outlined clearly as well as the most significant move away from the 'business-orientated' regime of the Conservative years to the Labour Government of 1997, which tried to re-establish the NHS as a public service. Clinical governance, according to Pollock, was integral to this change and therefore was widely supported. Moreover, according to Pollock, clinical governance is here to stay and will grow in the years ahead.

The essential features of clinical governance, including research and development, are outlined and the responsibility of NHS trusts (echoing Knight & Hostick), for providing the wherewithal for staff to achieve evidence-based practice, is described.

From the management perspective, clinical governance has definitely 'made a difference' according to Pollock. This is reflected in a more organised approach to NHS trust work with business and committees being organised explicitly around the tenets of clinical governance. Pollock provides some excellent and specific examples of how clinical governance is influencing policy and practice. Clinical governance is a driver for change and even cultural change within the NHS in Scotland and Pollock is a worthy advocate.

Caring for children

In the first of the chapters to consider specific clinical areas, Gosia Brykczyńska explains how working with children widened the net of accountability to include responsible adults who could grant consent to professionals to provide care and treatment for their children and also the extension of paediatric nursing to care of the whole family. Brykczyñska's chapter draws on some of the medical and social work scandals which have paved the way for the introduction of clinical governance. Brykczyñska introduces the concepts of power and political action as aspects of the accountability of paediatric nurses – and, thereby, all nurses – using the example of the part paediatric nurses could play in ensuring purpose-built facilities within an NHS trust if the trust did not want to provide them. Children are easily marginalised in the health service because they have no voice of their own, according to Brykczyñska. However, her argument that they take up a very small proportion of the NHS budget in proportion to their numbers in the general population may be answered simply by the fact that they tend, on the whole, to be less ill than adults, especially older people.

Learning disabilities

Bob Gates, Mick Wolverson and Jane Wray consider learning disability nursing. People with learning disability are a particularly vulnerable group in terms of physical, sexual and financial abuse. The issues of accountability and clinical governance, therefore, are highly relevant in this area of nursing. The UK Government has set standards regarding the care of people with learning disability. Therefore, there are standards against which care can be measured and judged.

A major feature of working with people who have learning disabilities is institutionalisation: not only bricks and mortar, but ways of doing things, and this can be very hard to challenge in the era of clinical governance. For an area of nursing practice which is often seen to be on the margins of nursing itself, the code of practice and professional conduct produced by the NMC are probably more important in terms of client protection. Gates *et al.* delineate the various areas of practice which they see as coming under the umbrella of clinical governance and, in common with Brykczyñska in Chapter 8, they consider autonomy. Uniquely, however, they consider advocacy. Implementing clinical governance in learning disability nursing poses some unique challenges and one of these is the number of agencies involved, such as social work and voluntary organisations. As a solution to this a model, referred to as RAID, is presented as one way of approaching clinical governance in learning disability nursing.

Midwifery

Rosemary Mander distinguishes nursing from midwifery and reckons that midwifery could learn a great deal from the nursing literature about accountability because it is not covered to any great extent in the midwifery literature. Perhaps this is because midwives take a certain degree of autonomy, and therefore accountability, for granted. Whatever the answer, both nurses and midwives will have a great deal to learn from Mander's chapter. Mander considers some definitions of accountability and examines how these apply to midwifery. Accountability to the employer, the woman and the profession are all considered. However, Mander reckons that personal accountability is the highest form of accountability. The historical development of accountability in midwifery is traced briefly and this complements the historical account of accountability in nursing presented by McGann in her chapter.

The issue of autonomy, one which is important in midwifery, is examined in some detail by Mander in terms of its relationship to accountability. Where accountability may appear to constrain the midwife, autonomy is a 'liberating phenomenon' and is regarded more positively. She mentions the interesting issue of 'attitudinal autonomy', which is really about the self-confidence to practice and to be accountable. Mander concludes by bringing clinical governance into the equation and her assessment is none too positive. She describes clinical governance as reductionist and likely to downgrade practice and this echoes many of the issues raised in Chapter 3.

Community nursing

Sarah Baggaley and Alison Bryans view community nursing mainly from a health visiting perspective. Recent political changes in the UK have brought community nursing more to the fore. This is set in the context of devolution in Scotland, where a more radical approach has been taken, especially in public health, against a background of poor health and life expectancy.

Changing skill mix, with an emphasis on saving money through the employment of lower grades of community nurses, has been a feature of community nursing. However, research has demonstrated the value of higher grades of community nurses with experience and the ability to delegate appropriately to lower grades. Delegation as part of team working is an essential feature of community nursing, but the NMC makes it clear where accountability lies when care has been delegated: with the registered nurse who does the delegating, who must ensure that adequate supervision is provided.

Nurses are attracted to working in the community due to greater levels of autonomy and professional accountability. The advent of clinical supervision has provided a framework within which quality patient care can be delivered and accountability ensured.

Clinical governance is as relevant to community nursing as any other area of nursing and Baggaley and Bryans discuss the implications for nurses in the community and the specifics of clinical effectiveness and evidence-based practice. The ability of health visitors to evaluate and implement research for practice, for example, will require investment of time and resources by managers.

Other developments, such as the renewed interest in public health nursing and nurse prescribing, are covered, as is the importance of patients' views. Despite all the changes which have taken place recently, Baggaley & Bryans are able to conclude in the same way: community nursing is challenging and satisfying and issues of accountability remain at the heart of practice

Mental health nursing

Stephen Tilley reflects upon the influence that clinical governance may have had upon accountability in mental heath nursing. The major change, since 1995, is that the introduction of clinical governance has put evidence-based practice at the heart of clinical practice. While Tilley and others acknowledge the accountability of nurses, including mental health nurses, towards managers and the health service, clinical governance may have shifted the balance, in the eyes of managers, towards serving the needs of the health service rather than the needs of patients. The 'Janus' nature of nurses, facing both ways at once, towards managers and patients, is a theme which Tilley expounds, and the NMC would appear to be supporting the notion that nursing practice is the delivery of evidence-based practice. In other words, nurses may face both ways at once but it is accountability to management which is taking precedence.

The consequences for accountability of new technology and the increasing move towards computerised records are considered. While computerised, integrated records fit neatly into the 'ideology' of clinical governance in that these records will be used to judge quality, the problematic issue of other forms of accountability – those interstitial aspects of care which may be accounted for informally by professionals and between professions – may go unrecorded.

The Government increasingly sees the views of patients as important in the planning and implementation of healthcare and this appears to imply that nurses must increasingly take into account users' views in practice and in their accounts of work. However, how this squares with the work of mental health nurses working with those detained against their will or how it squares with the use of the best available evidence, given current debates about nurses', including academic nurses', understanding of research and evidence production, remain problematic in exercising patient-centred care.

Tilley includes a moving extract from the autobiography of the father of evidence-based medicine, Archie Cochrane, which challenges many of the notions of this paradigm. Even Cochrane could see the limitations of applying a preconceived notion to a situation in which a patient was clearly suffering. The relief of the suffering came, not through the application of evidence but in acting in such a way – with compassion – that the reason for the suffering became apparent.

Research

Nursing and midwifery research are less new than they used to be but are still relatively new compared with other disciplines. Nursing research incorporating midwifery research, has fared very badly in UK national research assessment exercises sponsored by the higher education funding bodies. Nevertheless, the challenge remains to find a research base for our practice and this research must be as rigorous as research in any other field. One aspect of this rigour is the framework of accountability within which nursing and midwifery research must operate. There is accountability to funding bodies, to the NHS, to professional bodies and to the public. Furthermore, the introduction of research governance within health and social research has strengthened this framework of accountability.

Alison Tierney wrote the original chapter and the second editor joined her in writing the present chapter. The need for proper funding for nursing (and allied health professions) research has been recognised by the UK Departments of Health and by the higher education funding councils. Therefore, the future looks brighter than it ever did for nursing and midwifery research, but this means that both professions will have to be more aware of the constraints of accountability in research. This is a task which must be addressed by those providing undergraduate and postgraduate research courses for nursing and midwifery students.

Conclusion

Accountability remains a key topic and clinical governance has become a key topic for the professions of nursing and midwifery. The editors, apart from their own chapters, now hand over to the other authors for their accounts of how these are played out in their areas of responsibility, including those such as McGann, Jacobs and Tingle who offer views from other disciplinary perspectives.

This book was commissioned prior to the creation of the NMC, which succeeded the UKCC and the National Boards for Nursing in the four countries of the UK. The concept of accountability was first raised by the UKCC in 1989 and was subsequently incorporated into codes of practice in 1992 and 1996. The NMC produced a *Code of Professional Conduct* in 2002 which largely incorporates all of the existing codes of practice of the UKCC. Authors have referred to both codes of conduct (UKCC and NMC) in support of points throughout this text, representing the recent historical development of accountability and the relatively recent creation of the NMC. For clarity, with the permission of the NMC, we reproduce their 2002 *Code of Conduct* as an appendix to the text.

Chapter 2
The Development of Nursing as an Accountable Profession

Susan McGann

Introduction

The modern concept of professional accountability, applied to nursing, assumes that the nurse is a member of a profession. It depends on individual nurses being aware of their membership of a profession and accepting that status, with the rights and responsibilities that go with it (White, 1977). With the passing of the Nurses' Registration Acts, in 1919, nurses in Britain achieved the status of an accountable profession. This meant that registered nurses were legally accountable for their work and could be struck off the register for unprofessional behaviour. However, the concept of professional accountability is more intangible than legal accountability. In order for it to flourish, nurses had to become strong in their own professional self-esteem. This did not happen after 1919. Before considering why, we must look at the development of professional awareness among nurses.

Historical perspective

The year 1887 was the turning point in the emergence of nursing as a profession. In this year the first professional organisation for nurses was founded, the British Nurses' Association (BNA), and this marked the point when British nurses set their sights on professional status. It was inevitable that, sooner or later, efforts would be made to standardise the training of nurses and professional consciousness would emerge, but it took another 30 years before the majority of nurses in Britain realised the need for a professional organisation. Once nurses had joined a professional association in large numbers, they achieved state registration. The years between 1887 and 1919 were a period of professionalisation for nurses everywhere, which reflected the growth of the women's movement in North America and the suffrage campaign in Britain (Benson, 1990).

By the end of the nineteenth century, hospitals were no longer seen as charitable institutions for the sick poor but places where scientific medicine and surgery were practised, and they began to attract more patients, including the middle classes. The corresponding growth in the number of hospital beds depended on an increasing number of nurses to work in the hospitals. There was also an expansion of the nurse's duties, as the 'trained' nurse evolved in response to the advances in medicine. Nurses at the end of the nineteenth century were performing tasks – such as taking temperatures – which 20 years earlier no doctor would have delegated to them (Morten, 1895). These two related factors, the advances in medicine and the expansion in the number of hospital beds, produced a sharp rise in the number of nurse training schools in the country (Baly, 1986, p. 205).

The matrons of the time were aware of the rapid changes that were taking place in nursing and the uncontrolled nature of the development (Fenwick, 1897; Stewart, 1905). By 1886 the development of nursing was such that the Hospitals' Association (HA) appointed a committee to consider the possibility of establishing a register of nurses. Against the advice of the nurse members, the committee decided to set the standard for a registered nurse at one year's training. The matrons resigned from the Association and founded the BNA in 1887, the first professional association for nurses.

The British Nurses' Association

The founders of the BNA were predominantly educated, middle-class women who had entered nursing in the 1860s and 1870s, under the inspiration of Florence Nightingale's work (McGann, 1992). They had received little in the way of formal training and having risen to the top of the nursing world, as matrons of large teaching hospitals, they were imbued with the spirit of pioneers. They had seen nurses develop from being the 'handy-woman' of the 1850s and 1860s into the trained nurse with three years' systematic training in a hospital, able to share in the intellectual side of medicine. They saw nursing as an opportunity to improve society and as an area where an intelligent woman could make a career for herself. They had no doubt that the work of nurses was of such importance to the community that it required a system of registration. This would protect the public from the untrained nurse and it would protect the trained nurse from the competition of untrained women.

Mrs Bedford Fenwick

This group of matrons, who became the leaders of the movement to professionalise nursing, was led by Mrs Bedford Fenwick, a former matron of St Bartholomew's Hospital, and Isla Stewart, her successor there. Following the example of the medical profession, which was their natural role model and which had achieved state registration in 1858, they set out to achieve state registration for nurses. They were determined to set the standard for registration as high as the best nurses, in other words, three years' training, and believed that the only way to achieve this was by establishing a statutory system of registration, since a voluntary system would never reach the poorer hospitals. Mrs Fenwick outlined the requirements of a nurses' registration act to the first meeting of the BNA. The act would set up a general nursing council (GNC), which would be a legally recognised body. This council, composed largely of the heads of the nursing profession, would be responsible for setting the standard of training, examination and registration (Fenwick, 1887).

The leaders of the campaign for state registration realised that one of the keys to professional status was the education of nurses. Owing to the rapid evolution of nurses' training schools, the majority were schools only in name (Fenwick, 1897). Each hospital had developed its own system of training in isolation. Standards varied greatly, from the big teaching hospitals at one end of the scale to the small cottage hospitals at the other end. As a result of this 'free for all', the term 'trained' nurse could mean anything. The progressives regarded the introduction of a uniform system of training, followed by a standard examination, as a priority (Stewart, 1895). They wanted to remove the uncertainty and ambiguity of the position of the trained nurse:

> We are fully determined that, in the future, the public shall know as precisely what is meant by a trained nurse as what is meant by a qualified medical man, and the nurse's right to her title, free from the intrusion of unqualified women, shall be as unquestioned as his.   (Mollett, 1898)

In her speech to the International Council of Nurses' Congress in 1901, Mrs Fenwick enumerated the profession's most pressing needs: preliminary education before entering the hospital wards; postgraduate teaching to keep abreast of developments; instruction as nurse teachers; a state-constituted board to examine and maintain discipline; and legal status to protect their professional rights and to ensure professional autonomy. She saw the choice facing nurses clearly:

> We stand now at the Rubicon . . . we must either go forward or go back . . . before us lies the organised and scientific profession of our dreams, in which every duly qualified nurse is registered as a skilled practitioner. Behind us is that dreary downhill path, descending to a disorganised vocation of obsolete methods, in the ranks of which all kinds and conditions of workers, good, bad and indifferent, struggle and compete.
>
> (Fenwick, 1901a)

The campaign for the state registration of nurses divided the hospital and nursing world into two camps. Those who were in favour of professional autonomy for nurses supported the campaign; those who did not want to see nursing become a profession opposed it. The opposition numbered among its members many influential persons from the medical and hospital establishment and, from the nursing establishment itself, no less a figure than Florence Nightingale. Miss Nightingale was opposed to any system of public registration for nurses (Stewart, 1895; Cook, 1913, pp. 359–60). She considered that it could only mislead the public into thinking that a registered nurse was a good nurse, whereas the qualities of a good nurse were just those qualities which could never be judged by a theoretical examination. She opposed all attempts to professionalise nursing, believing that nursing was a vocation and an art, and should only be followed by those who had a 'calling' (Cook, 1913, pp. 2, 269).

Eva Luckes, the matron of the London Hospital, shared Miss Nightingale's views about nursing and the two women became friends through their shared opposition to state registration. Miss Luckes regretted the growing tendency among nurses and the public to overrate both the importance and the amount of technical knowledge that a nurse should possess. She believed the human side of a nurse's work would always be more important: 'People too frequently forget that nursing is an Art . . . nursing must not be regarded merely as a profession' (Luckes, 1914, p. 3).

Professional registration

In 1892 the British Nurses' Association, which had been granted the prefix 'Royal' (RBNA), announced its intention to apply for a royal charter authorising it to form a register of trained nurses. The opponents of registration feared that this would give the RBNA undue influence over nurses. The issue became one of intense public debate, with both sides lobbying in support of their case. In the end, the Privy Council steered a middle course. The charter was granted but it did not empower the RBNA to set up a register of trained nurses who could call themselves 'registered' or 'chartered'. Instead, it could maintain 'a list of persons who may have applied to have their names entered therein as nurses' (Cook, 1913, p. 364).

Matrons' Council of Great Britain and Ireland

Following this success, the opponents of registration gained control of the RBNA. Membership was also open to doctors, and when the Association was founded many eminent physicians and surgeons had been invited to join. Under the terms of the new charter, they were able to gain control and remove Mrs Fenwick from the council. Two years later, they succeeded in carrying a vote against registration.

This experience was not wasted on nursing leaders, as it brought home to them the strength of feeling of the opposition to state registration for nurses. They realised that any attempt to promote the status of nursing would arouse 'prehistoric prejudices' and 'a multitude of vested interests' (Dock, 1899, 1901). At the International Council of Nurses' Congress, in 1901, Catherine Wood, former Lady Superintendent of Great Ormond Street Hospital and one of the founders of the RBNA, spoke of the lessons they had learnt:

> In England we have tried the experiment of organising the profession in conjunction with the medical profession, but with disastrous results; it is

a failure . . . we must be free to organise ourselves; the relation of man to woman complicates the situation; the relative position of doctor and nurse makes it impossible. Though our work is in common, the details differ, and though we do not claim independence of the medical profession, we claim freedom to discuss our own affairs, to make our own laws, to decide on common principles of work.   (Wood, 1901)

After her expulsion from the RBNA Mrs Fenwick and Miss Stewart, who had resigned from the Association, founded the Matrons' Council of Great Britain and Ireland. Membership was restricted to matrons and superintendents of nurses, and the aim was to provide members with a forum for discussing professional issues. They were all agreed that the priority for the profession was a uniform system of training and state registration (Stewart, 1898). A strong influence on Mrs Fenwick at this time was the American women's movement. In 1892 she travelled to Chicago to organise the British nursing section at the World's Fair to be held there in 1893. This was very successful. The most long-lasting effects of her trips to Chicago, however, were her contact with Mrs May Wright Sewall, founder of the International Council of Women, and her friendship with Isabel Hampton Robb, the director of the Nursing Department at the Johns Hopkins Hospital in Baltimore, and her assistant Lavinia Dock. Robb and Dock were leading the move to professionalise nurses in the United States (James, 1979, p. 204).

Miss Robb and Mrs Fenwick seized the opportunity presented by the inclusion, for the first time, of a Women's Section at the World's Fair to publicise the new profession of nursing. They planned a conference on nursing, for which Miss Robb carefully chose a series of papers that illustrated the developments in nursing and the need for a higher standard of education. At the conference, Miss Robb spoke of the responsibility of hospitals to provide nurses with a real education in return for the nursing services rendered. She believed that the pioneer generation of schools was no longer good enough (James, 1979, p. 229).

When she returned from Chicago, Mrs Fenwick became involved in the organisation of the 1899 Congress of the International Council of Women, to be held in London. Once again she took the opportunity to organise a nursing section, which attracted a considerable number of foreign nurses. These delegates were invited to attend the annual meeting of the Matrons' Council, held the day after the Congress (McGann, 1992, pp. 41–2). The guest speaker at this meeting was Mrs May Wright Sewall, the President of the International Council of Women, who addressed the meeting on the subject of professional organisation:

One of the chief objects of organisation is to get professional recognition, to command the respect from the public, which you think you deserve. As an isolated individual you are unable to do it . . . when you come into your peerage you can establish laws which will govern your wages, and that will put you into a different attitude toward the public and the public will pay to each individual the respect it pays to the organisation.

(Sewall, 1905)

At this meeting Mrs Fenwick proposed the establishment of an International Council of Nurses (ICN), which would be organised on the same basis as the International Council of Women, membership being based on one national association to represent the nurses of each country. The ICN, which came into existence the following year, strengthened the efforts of nurses for professional improvement in all countries. It organised international congresses, which encouraged nurses to discuss questions of common interest and importance to their profession (Fenwick, 1901b). The leaders of the campaign to professionalise nursing valued these contacts with nurses in other countries. Mrs Fenwick's journal, *The Nursing Record and Hospital World*, renamed *The British Journal of Nursing* in 1902, became the official organ of the ICN and carried her ideas on the professional status of nurses around the world.

The Matrons' Council was concerned about the need to raise professional awareness among nurses in Britain. In the United States nurses had followed the example of university graduates and started to form alumnae associations. The first had been formed in 1891, and by 1897 the majority of training schools in the USA and Canada had them. These associations provided the nurses with a professional organisation, which could look after their social, economic, educational and professional interests. Following a paper by Miss Robb on the subject, to the Matrons' Council, Miss Stewart proposed the formation of the League of St Bartholomew's Nurses. The League, the first of its kind in this country, was inaugurated in December 1899 (McGann, 1992, pp. 67–8). Over the next ten years five more Leagues were formed, based on training schools, and in 1904 a National Council of Nurses was set up, composed of delegates from the existing nurses' societies and associations, to represent British nurses in the International Council of Nurses.

Political perspective

The process of professionalisation of nurses continued in the years leading up to World War I. At an international level, the ICN held meetings and congresses in Berlin in 1904, in Paris in 1907, in London in 1909 and in Cologne in 1912. For nurses campaigning for professional status and registration against prejudice and apathy in their own countries, the international meetings were of the greatest value: 'It is an inspiration and source of encouragement to know that other countries are facing the same problems, working towards the same common standards' (Robb, 1909).

In the early years of the twentieth century, the campaigners had reason to be optimistic about achieving state registration. In 1902 a Midwives Act was passed, establishing a Central Midwives Board and introducing the registration of midwives in England. In 1905, a Select Committee of the House of Commons reported in favour of state registration for nurses, and the following year the British Medical Association (BMA) voted almost unanimously in favour of state registration for nurses. Nurses were achieving legal status in other countries: first in South Africa in 1891, when the Cape Medical Council took on the responsibility for registering trained nurses; then in Natal in 1899, in New Zealand in 1901, in four states in the United States in 1903, and in the Transvaal in 1906. By 1914, 40 of the American States and the Scandinavian countries had state registration of nurses (*British Journal of Nursing*, 1903; *Nursing Times*, 1921).

Early registration bill

In Britain, the first bill for the registration of nurses was introduced to Parliament in 1904 as a Private Member's bill. It had been drawn up by Mrs Fenwick and Miss Stewart, with the assistance of Dr Bedford Fenwick, who fully supported his wife's campaign for the professional status of nurses. They had formed the Society for the State Registration of Nurses in 1902, to lead the campaign for registration. A second Private Member's bill for the registration of nurses was introduced in Parliament in 1904 on behalf of the RBNA. Although it was now promoting a bill for the registration of nurses, it was, in Mrs Fenwick's words, an employers' bill, giving the controlling vote on the proposed GNC to hospital and medical authorities. The bill drafted by the Fenwicks gave a majority of the seats on the proposed council to nurses, thus ensuring that nurses had professional autonomy.

It was at this point that the Select Committee of the House of Commons was appointed to inquire into the subject. The Committee heard evidence from witnesses representing the medical and nursing professions, and from lay people, including Dr and Mrs Bedford Fenwick, Isla Stewart and Miss Luckes. The Committee reported in favour of state registration and accepted that three years was the most practical period for the training of a nurse. The pro-registration party were confident that statutory recognition of their profession could no longer be postponed, but they slowly realised that the Government had no plans to draw up a nurses' registration bill. When the two Private Members' bills for registration were reintroduced in the House of Commons, they were defeated.

A third bill for registration was promoted in 1908, this time in the House of Lords. This bill proposed an 'official directory' of nurses, instead of a legal system of registration, and was promoted by the opponents of professional autonomy for nurses. The bill made no provision for a minimum standard of training or for a GNC. Mrs Fenwick described it as 'the Nurses' Enslavement Bill', and its defeat was interpreted as a sign of support for the cause of state registration. The Fenwicks' bill was then introduced in the Lords and was passed but, once again, without Government support, it failed to get a reading in the Commons.

A feeling of frustration set in among the leaders of the campaign for registration in 1909, after a delegation to the Prime Minister had failed to obtain any guarantee of support for registration. A decision was taken to form a Central Committee for the State Registration of Nurses, which would represent the eight existing associations of trained nurses in the country, to promote a joint bill. The bill incorporated the three principles, which Mrs Fenwick regarded as beyond compromise: a minimum standard of three years' training as the qualification for registration; a uniform curriculum and examination for all nurses; and the appointment of a general nursing council to be responsible for professional standards.

This joint bill was introduced in the House of Commons, as a Private Members' bill, in 1910, and each year after that up to 1914, but failed to get a hearing. Miss Dock remarked: 'There are those who believe that no woman's bill will seem important to the House of Commons until women are fully enfranchised' (Dock, 1912, p. 59). Mrs Fenwick shared this view: as a suffragist for many years she believed that the nurses' campaign for legal recognition was part of women's struggle for the right to professional status and autonomy. This view was given weight by the fact that the opposition was not against registration in itself: it had in fact proposed several systems of registration over the years, but would oppose any system of registration that gave nurses legal status and professional autonomy.

The Government argued that they could not afford to ignore the opponents of registration, and there is no doubt that the opponents commanded real influence. But, as Miss Stewart said in 1905, the real enemies of registration were the rank and file of nurses, numbering ostensibly 70 000 or 80 000, who through their apathy allowed the Government to do nothing (Stewart, 1905). The number of nurses who supported state registration through membership of one of the nurses' organisations, estimated at 10 000, was a small minority of the total number of nurses in the country. When World War I started in 1914, the Central Committee's bill for state registration had just received a majority at its first reading in the House of Commons, but had been refused a second reading. With the outbreak of war, the facility to promote Private Members' bills was suspended.

The war

The war saw the mobilisation of thousands of nurses. Over 10 000 joined the regular army nursing service, Queen Alexandra's Imperial Military Nursing Service, and saw action at the front (Haldane, 1923). Through the Territorial Army Nursing Service approximately 6000 nurses were employed in the temporary military hospitals at home and abroad (McGann, 1992, pp. 88–96). Another 6000 nurses were deployed, through the British Red Cross Society (BRCS) in the auxiliary hospitals at home and abroad. Finally, there were over 12 000 VADs, the untrained women who worked as nurses through the Voluntary Aid Detachments run by the BRCS.

At the start of the war the Government had delegated responsibility for the organisation of the voluntary medical and nursing services to the BRCS. The nursing profession was dismayed that after 20 years of campaigning for the professional status of trained nurses, the Government still regarded nursing as philanthropic work. In the first five months of the war, from August to December of 1914, many auxiliary hospitals were set up by wealthy ladies with no nursing experience. The National Council of Trained Nurses placed on record its disapproval of the nursing of sick and wounded soldiers in military and auxiliary hospitals by 'untrained and unskilled women' (*British Journal of Nursing*, 1915a). This was an attack on the VADs and the amateur hospitals which had been encouraged by the BRCS.

By the beginning of 1915, the unorganised state of nursing was beginning to cause problems. The Government found it necessary to tighten up the issue of passports to nurses going to work abroad. It had been found that many women volunteering for nursing work abroad were untrained, and on arrival at their destination were an embarrassment to the authorities. Sarah Swift, as the Matron-in-Chief of the BRCS, had the job of checking the qualifications of all the nurses volunteering for work at home and abroad. In 1915 she also became responsible for interviewing and selecting VADs who volunteered for nursing (McGann, 1992, pp. 167–9).

The nursing profession had advised from the start that these untrained women should only be allowed to nurse in the auxiliary hospitals, and then under the supervision of trained nurses. By the spring of 1915 there was such a shortage of nurses that it became necessary to allow the VADs to work in the wards of military hospitals, albeit again under supervision. Mrs Fenwick pointed out that, had registration been introduced before the war, the shortage of nurses would have been foreseen and a register of nurses would have been available to check their qualifications and to provide a means of communicating with trained nurses (*British Journal of Nursing*, 1915b).

By the end of 1915, Miss Swift had come to the conclusion that the unorganised state of nursing was 'chaos', and in no one's interest, least of all nurses'. She felt that to wait until after the war for a system of state registration would be too late, as by that time thousands of VADs would be competing with trained nurses. She thought the profession should organise itself on a voluntary basis. She proposed the establishment of a College of Nursing, to be run by nurses with the cooperation of the training schools. The College would introduce a uniform curriculum of training and recognise approved training schools, grant certificates and maintain a register of nurses who had received these certificates.

She enlisted the support of Arthur Stanley (the Chairman of the BRCS and, as Treasurer of St Thomas' Hospital, an influential person among hospital governors) and three eminent matrons, Alicia Lloyd Still (St Thomas' Hospital), Rachel Cox-Davies (Royal Free Hospital) and Miss Haughton (Guy's Hospital). They wrote to the matrons and managers of the large teaching hospitals around the country proposing the scheme for a College of Nursing and asking for their support. After three months of discussions the College was launched in April 1916, with the support of the training schools (McGann, 1992, pp. 170–80).

The old state registration party was opposed to the College of Nursing. They believed that it was only a matter of time before the Government accepted the necessity for state registration and they were not prepared to accept a voluntary system. Mrs Fenwick, in particular, would not countenance the involvement of hospital managers in the professional affairs of nurses. For many years her vision had been of an independent nursing profession, governed by an independent general nursing council. Prolonged negotiations between the promoters of the College and the state registration party took place. They all recognised that conditions had changed since before the war, and that the time was right for a new initiative. Many of the old campaigners were won over when the founders of the College agreed to make a bill for state registration a priority.

The membership of the College of Nursing grew rapidly, despite the fact that the war was still going on and nurses were scattered all over the country and abroad. By the end of 1916 there were 2000 members; by the end of 1917 the number was 8000, and by 1919 it had reached 13 000. The rank and file of nurses were joining a professional organisation for the first time. The Council of the College attempted to reach agreement with the Central Committee for the State Registration of Nurses over a joint bill. Negotiations finally broke down in 1918, and the two groups promoted separate bills, the Central Committee's in the House of Commons and the College's in the Lords.

Registration Act 1919

A majority of the profession was now agreed on the need for registration and the Government appears to have accepted registration in principle at this point (Abel-Smith, 1960, p. 93). The Minister of Health, Dr Addison, negotiated with the College and the Central Committee in an attempt to reach an agreed bill, but when this proved impossible he asked the two parties to withdraw their bills and promised a Government bill. This was introduced in Parliament in November 1919, and became law in December. Separate Acts for Scotland and Ireland were passed. After a campaign of over 30 years, nurses in Britain had achieved the status of an accountable profession.

There are several reasons why the Government was prepared to give nurses state registration in 1919 and not before. The opposition from within the profession had disappeared: Florence Nightingale had died in 1910 and Miss Luckes died in February 1919. Nurses were becoming more politicised: 20 000 had joined the College of Nursing between 1916 and 1920. The opposition from the medical profession and hospital governors had been won over by giving them a consultative role in the College of Nursing.

In the wider world of politics the registration of nurses, like women's suffrage, was no longer a football for party politics, which it had been before the war. The status of women had benefited from their war work and the principle of female suffrage had been accepted when women over 30 were given the vote in 1918. Some Members of Parliament feared the growing industrial unrest would spread to women workers. During the war the number of women joining trade unions had increased sharply. There was also the threat that if state registration was withheld any longer, nurses would be driven into the arms of the Labour Party, who had made an issue of their poor wages and conditions (Dingwall *et al.*, 1988, pp. 86–7).

Conclusions

Like the achievement of women's suffrage, registration did not prove to be the turning point in the profession's progress (Carter, 1939). The 'battle of the nurses' for and against registration had ended in the compromise of the 1919 Nurses' Registration Acts. Unlike the Midwives Act of 1902, the Nurses' Registration Acts did not give nurses legal status, and nursing by unregistered women calling themselves nurses was not prohibited. This created a second grade of nurse outside the control of the three General Nursing Councils (England and Wales, Scotland, and Ireland). In addition to the register for general nurses, the Acts had set up five supplementary registers. These were for male nurses, mental nurses, nurses of 'mental defectives', sick children's nurses and fever nurses. This was professionally divisive and prevented the development of a comprehensive general training scheme.

Mrs Fenwick believed at first that having won a two-thirds majority of nurses on the GNC, they had secured professional autonomy. However, her vision of a nursing profession equal in status to the medical profession was not to be. The Government had designed that the Act was 'confined within the smallest possible compass' (Dingwall *et al.*, 1988, p. 88), and all the decisions of the GNC were subject to the approval of the Minister of Health and of both Houses of Parliament. The first intervention came from Parliament, when the rules for the registration of existing nurses, drawn up by the Council, were significantly altered by the Commons. The definition of 'existing nurse' was widened to include a level of experienced but untrained nurses that the majority of the profession considered unwise.

When the Council drafted a syllabus of training, based on the syllabus in use at the Nightingale School at St Thomas' Hospital, the Minister refused to make it compulsory. He considered that it demanded too high a standard of general education from probationers and was impractical for training schools. The syllabus remained advisory. Again, on the inspection of training schools, the Minister refused to ratify the scheme drawn up by the Council and, without any financial provision for inspectors, members of the

Council had to carry out limited inspections themselves (McGann, 1992, pp. 207–208). There was nothing in the Act to prohibit the training of nurses by training schools which had not been approved by the Council.

The power of the profession through the General Nursing Councils to raise professional standards was very limited. The educational standards the nurse leaders had set out to achieve through state registration were diluted or obstructed by both the Government and Parliament. Any attempt by the Councils to improve the standard of training was weighed against the cost implications for the hospitals. By 1920 the hospitals had become totally dependent on the provision of cheap nursing services provided by the nurse training schools. The hospitals were running on deficit budgets by this time and a threat to the supply of nursing recruits would make matters worse. The apprenticeship system of training, evolved to deal with the conditions in the nineteenth-century hospitals, was out of date but hospital economics depended on its survival (Baly, 1986, p. 223).

This system of training, with its emphasis on discipline and conformity, produced nurses who were obedient and uncritical (Helmstadter, 1993). On top of this, the hierarchical organisation of nursing in hospitals produced a hierarchy of accountability, which detracted from the accountability of the nurse at the lowest level. Without legal status, without professional autonomy and with a system of training which undermined professional confidence it was unlikely that nurses in Britain would develop that professional *esprit de corps* which was necessary to foster professional accountability.

Chapter 3

Accountability and Clinical Governance in Nursing: a Critical Overview of the Topic

Kerry Jacobs

Accountability is a complex, elusive and multi-faceted concept. It does not lend itself to neat, self-contained definitions, although this has not prevented the proliferation of these. (Pyper, 1996, p. 1)

Introduction

Accountability is one of those delightfully paradoxical words because nobody is sure what it means. More accountability is self-evidently a good thing and something to be encouraged by the public, professions and the State. However, exactly how to deliver this accountability eludes everybody and the question of why accountability should make us all better off is never asked. Inevitably the term is captured by different interests and ideologies. The State wants inspection and control; nurses want self-development, increased autonomy and improved professional status; management want cost control and predictability; while the public want to know why they do not have personal one-to-one nursing 24 hours a day and the latest medical technology (after all, they do pay their taxes).

Therefore, a simple definition of accountability becomes meaningless. To complicate the issue further the term accountability doesn't exist in many languages. This is true in German, Italian and, as noted by Melia (1995), in Spanish. When translating we are forced to turn to words like responsibility, answerability and even reporting. At best the term accountability is an Anglo-Saxon one most commonly used in English speaking countries such as the US and the UK. Therefore, it is clear that the term accountability is contingent, contestable and confusing.

However, within nursing research and practice the issue of accountability is an important one. The conflicting and contradictory concepts associated with accountability in nursing can be found reflected in the introduction to Watson (1995). He starts by identifying the concept of accountability with the purchaser-provider distinction in the NHS and then goes on to present Prentice's suggestion (1994) that accountability was 'answering, responsiveness, openness . . . not to mention participation and obedience to external laws'. According to Watson accountability is something hierarchical, structural and institutional; something about markets, reporting and performance measurement.

However, it is also evident that the concept of accountability is intrinsically linked to the concept of professionalism. Watson (1992) suggests that accountability is the very essence of professionalism. Nurses are accountable to the general public for their practice. However, in practice this does not involve giving an account to the public or to patients but rather registration (and possibly regulation) by a professional body – the Nursing and Midwifery Council (NMC). According to Watson (1992) accountability is defined as a feature of professionalism and is understood as 'answering' to an external governing body rather than to an employer or to patients. To extend this understanding accountability can be seen as a characteristic, or trait, identified by authors such as Wilensky (1964) and Millerson (1964), which distinguishes professions from non-professions. Therefore, for nursing, the concept of accountability becomes a rhetorical device in the argument over whether nursing is or isn't a profession within the framework of theories of professionalisation (or perhaps deprofessionalisation).

Central to a discussion of accountability in nursing, and to Watson (1995), was the work of Batey & Lewis (1982) and Lewis & Batey (1982). However, these papers are fundamentally flawed. They failed to engage with the literature on organisations, power, accountability and control. Batey & Lewis lack a concept of power, import a moral order (rightful/legitimate) without indicating a source and reduce nursing to moral conventionality. They fail to recognise that nursing autonomy and discretion are a reflection of power and only make sense in a given context. They also confuse freedom and control as they conclude that 'The principal consequence of autonomy is accountability' (p. 17). They fail to see that in an organisational context it is the absence or limitation of autonomy that gives rise to accountability obligations, that reflect relationships of power and control. The very organisational structure that they suggest fosters autonomy is explicitly and fundamentally designed to reduce it (Emmanuel *et al.*, 1990; Anthony & Govindarajan, 1998).

Lewis & Batey carry forward and compound many of the mistakes made in the earlier paper. It is only halfway through this second paper that they admit that they have limited their discussions to structural definitions of accountability (presumably a limitation also applying to the earlier paper), thereby invalidating the good and interesting work on accountability done by earlier authors and their own empirical evidence, which clearly shows that accountability can be understood in a much broader sense. The nursing directors they interviewed suggested that accountability was associated with a personal commitment, a professional disposition, commitment to a set of values and being 'true to yourself'. Their informants indicate that accountability can be seen as 'dues-paying' and that it is connected with the relationships between nurses and hospital administrators and between nurses and doctors. This evidence indicates that there is an important power element in their own findings, which they ignore.

In reviewing Lewis & Batey it is clear that their understanding of accountability was fundamentally confused on a number of key points. They criticise recounting and suggest that accounting (or perhaps accountability) has no time restriction. However, in the literature on accounting and accountability these things are universally seen as *ex post facto*. It is only possible to account for an action after the action. Lewis & Batey subsequently contradict their earlier point with the quote that 'to be accountable is to be answerable for what one has done, to stand behind one's decisions and actions' (p. 11). It is difficult to see how one could 'stand behind' something that has not yet occurred. Therefore, their position is internally contradictory and their distinction between recounting and accounting meaningless.

A second major flaw in Lewis & Batey is their confusion over the nature of control. They suggest that it is fallacious reasoning to equate accountability with control. Accountability and control are not the same thing and authors such as Passos (1973) who have suggested this are wrong. Well, all that can be said is that Lewis & Batey are wrong, and that they are inconsistent with their own structuralist/functionalist worldview. Essentially if structural accountability is not a form of control what is it? Within control theory accountability can operate at any stage of the process as a form of feedback or feed-forward and is one important element of a system of control. An individual can be accountable for their use of inputs according to some specified rules, for following procedural guidelines and for the achievement or non-achievement of specified outputs (Emmanuel *et al.*, 1990; Anthony & Govindarajan, 1998).

In fact the form of control depends upon the point (inputs, process or outputs) at which it is appropriate and possible to account (Ouchi, 1979). Although Lewis & Batey do not acknowledge that accountability is part of control they contradict their own assertion and suggest that accountability can 'support tight *control* over nursing service goals and functions' (p. 13, italics added) and illustrate the basic concept of control by suggesting that accountability structures make the purposes, processes and outcomes of nursing visible to those in power. Therefore Lewis & Batey can be seen to be internally inconsistent. They contradict their earlier statement that accountability and control are not linked with an almost perfect illustration of the link between accountability, control and power. It is just a pity that they did not recognise or develop this link.

How then is the concept of accountability seen and defined by the nursing profession? Is this consistent with Lewis & Batey's confused structuralism? For nurses in the UK the central concept of accountability is set out in the *Code of Professional Conduct* (NMC, 2002b). A more extensive discussion of the issue of accountability is to be found in the earlier document – the *Guidelines for Professional Practice* (UKCC, 1996a) where the UKCC commented on and explained the accountability obligations contained in the then *Code of Professional Practice*. The NMC code is heavily based on the earlier UKCC guidelines.

The NMC define 'accountable' as 'responsible for something or to someone' (NMC, 2002b, p. 10). The earlier UKCC guidelines extended this and suggested that nurses have three accountability obligations: a professional accountability, a contractual accountability to the employer and accountability at law for their actions. However, the core of all of the elements of a nurse's accountability is a sense of personal accountability. This personal accountability is reflected in the NMC Code as follows: As a registered nurse, midwife or health visitor, you are personally accountable for your practice (NMC, 2002b).

Ultimately each nurse must answer for his or her own actions. The NMC pointedly suggest that it is no defence to suggest that you were acting on someone else's orders. If the work is delegated to someone who is not registered with the NMC, the nurse's 'accountability' is to make sure that this person is suitably competent and supervised.

The accountability obligations contained in the NMC Code can be grouped around a central theme – an obligation or duty of care to patients. The idea that nurses should put the interests of patients and colleagues prior to their own interests is also reinforced with the injunctions that they should maintain their professional knowledge and skills, assist others in their professional development, recognise their own limitations, work cooperatively with patients and colleagues, report any conscientious objections and any circumstances which may compromise standards of care and endanger patients and/or colleagues, not abuse their privileged position or exploit their professional status for financial gain and maintain confidentiality.

Evidently, the NMC, and UKCC before it, use the term accountability to mean a number of things. First and foremost is the idea of personal accountability. This concept is taken to mean that the responsibility for patient care cannot be delegated to another person (either upward to senior staff or downward to unregistered staff). Ultimately each nurse must (or must be able to) answer for his/her own actions. However, to whom they have to answer remains undefined: the NMC, colleagues, management or themselves.

This ambiguity and the suggestion of a personal accountability based on a personal set of values imply a different understanding of accountability. Accountability is a fidelity to a personal set of values, based on the core values outlined by the NMC, in particular the obligation to protect and care for patients. In exercising this personal accountability the nurse may have to weigh up conflicting demands and needs and be prepared to justify their decision. While this could possibly involve giving an account to colleagues or to the NMC, this is mostly about accounting to one self.

This concept of professional accountability being a personal accountability is also found in Clark (2000), which was one of the key papers from the Second WHO Ministerial conference on Nursing and Midwifery in

Europe. Although Clark adopted the Lewis & Batey definition of account-ability (formal obligation to disclose to others . . .) she defined professional accountability as follows:

> Professional accountability means that the professional takes a decision or action not because someone has told him or her to do so, but because, having weighed up the alternatives and consequences in the light of the best available knowledge, he or she believes that it is the right decision or action to take. (Clark, 2000, p. 2)

Clark continues by arguing that this involves the nurse being able to 'account for' their action but this is not in a formal or structural sense. Essentially the action of professional accountability is an action of professional judgement where the nurse may be called to justify their decision but the primary test is their own values and conscience – what they believe is right.

The NMC (2002), UKCC (1996a), Clark (2000) and Watson (1995) acknowledge that nurses are obliged to 'account' to other bodies and indi-viduals. Watson (1995) lists patients and families, management, educational institutions and the medical profession. Through the delegation of budgets nurses are accountable to non-nurses for their actions and their use of resources. The fact that budgets are inherently a form of control and there-fore a source of power is implicitly acknowledged. Nursing practice is made visible and calculable through the technology of budgetary control, which is part of the hierarchy or structure of the organisation. Accountability is a form of structural or hierarchical control.

In terms of the relationship with the medical profession, nurses 'appear' to have gained some measure of autonomy and independence. For example, they now have the power to administer intravenous medication and there has been a long ongoing discussion over whether nurses should or shouldn't have prescribing rights. However, many aspects of the practice of nursing remain firmly under the authority and supervision of the medical profession. The administration of drugs remains under the imprimatur of a doctor's prescription. Nurses are, in effect, required to account to doctors for their clinical practice, for following their commands. Therefore accountability is about professional power, jurisdiction and subordination. Accountability is a reflection of power relations and control in a subordinated division of labour (Abbott, 1988, p. 73).

On a day-to-day basis nurses might be called to account by patients or family members and therefore be required to explain what they are doing and why. They may have to give an account of their practices or even of the practices of other clinical staff within the NHS. However, because this is infor-mal and nurses are not 'obliged' to be accountable to patients Watson (1992) suggests that this is being accountable 'for' rather than 'to' patients. Therefore, nurses aren't really accountable to patients. However, who nurses are 'accountable-for-patients' to remains undefined. Watson (1995) acknowledges that these concepts of accountability are complex, confused, contradictory and perhaps unhelpful to good nursing practice. The next section of this paper attempts to bring some clarity to the discussion by summarising theories and research pertaining to the issue of accountability.

Accountability

A number of authors have attempted to structure the concept of accountability. One of the standard distinctions is between political and managerial accountability. Day & Klein (1987) define political accountability as 'those with delegated authority being answerable for their actions to the people, whether directly in simple societies or indirectly in complex societies' and managerial accountability as 'making those with delegated authority answerable for carrying out agreed tasks' (p. 26).

Stewart (1984) presents a generally similar analysis but distinguishes between public, managerial and commercial accountability. He argues that there is a hierarchy or ladder of accountability, starting with accountability for probity and legality, going on to process accountability, performance accountability, programme accountability and finally policy accountability. He argues that the distinctive feature of public accountability is the concern for the 'higher' forms of accountability (programme and policy) while managerial accountability is generally concerned with the 'lower' forms (programme, performance and commercial accountability when the market can provide standards). However, these typologies are primarily concerned with what accountability should be rather than how accountability is understood. They therefore seem to be distant from an understanding of how the term accountability is understood in the context of nursing.

Sinclair offers a more useful framework. She recognises that the term accountability can be used to mean many different things, describing accountability as chameleon-like, multiple, fragmented and subject to continual reconstruction (Sinclair, 1995, p. 231). Her analysis of accountability was not based on a conceptual typology but on an empirical study of the views of chief executives in Australian public sector agencies. Rather than attempting to map 'real' forms of accountability she sought to describe how the term accountability was understood and used in practice. Based on this analysis she suggested that CEOs (chief executive officers) perceived five forms of accountability in the public sector – political, public, managerial, professional and personal. She utilised two different discourses in their discussion of accountability – structural and personal.

Sinclair suggested that political accountability was about straight-line relationships or chains of accountability, the accountability of the public servant to the minister and of the minister to parliament (and perhaps even parliament to the electorate). Public accountability was understood as the more informal but direct accountability to the public, interested communities and individuals. This includes public enquiries, newspaper reports, and agencies such as the ombudsman, the Auditor-General and Treasury.

Administrative, managerial or bureaucratic accountability were historically seen as the same thing, arising by virtue of a person's location within a hierarchy in which a superior calls to account a subordinate for the performance of delegated duties.

These aspects of accountability were evident in the structural analysis of Batey & Lewis, who argued that authority and therefore accountability was tied to position. However, Sinclair (p. 227) suggested that recent public sector reforms had led to a distinction between administrative and managerial accountability. Managerial accountability was seen as monitoring inputs and outputs or outcomes while administrative accountability was seen as being concerned with monitoring the processes by which inputs are transformed. In effect this fits the distinction between what Hood (1995) called New Public Management (NPM) and the pre-existing doctrines of public accountability and administration (Progressive Public Administration).

Sinclair suggested that professional accountability involved the sense of duty that one has as a member of a professional or expert group. However, this professional accountability was given very different meanings by different CEOs. For some CEOs professional accountability meant being the top professional in an agency dominated by a particular professional group; for others it meant being a professional administrator or manager; while for others being professionally accountable involved representing the professional values of the agency workforce to a sceptical government or community. Little mention was made of the fundamental idea of giving an account for action to a group of peers or to a professional association.

Personal accountability was described as fidelity to personal conscience in basic values such as respect for human dignity and acting in a manner that accepts responsibility for affecting the lives of others. Ultimately this was seen to rest on an internalised set of moral or ethical values. However, each of these forms could be articulated within two different discourses, structural and personal. Within a structural discourse accountability was an objectified feature of a contract or position: accountability was not problematic but could be 'delivered to' and 'extracted from' others by following procedure (Sinclair, 1995, p. 232). Again, this could be seen to be akin to the Batey & Lewis stance. However, within a personal discourse accountability was something that CEOs uphold and fear, something about which they feel both anguish and attachment as a moral practice (Sinclair, 1995, p. 232). Curiously enough this seems to be more characteristic of the Batey & Lewis empirics.

Sinclair develops the idea that there is a fundamental duality to the concept of accountability through her distinction between a structural and an individual discourse. However, this duality is not well explained or defined and needs further work. Munro & Mouritson (1996) explore the idea of duality by suggesting that accountability should be understood as a broad concept that extends beyond formal accounts to embrace concepts of how individuals give account of and for their daily lives and, in doing so, produce and reproduce their individual and collective identities. To further explore the idea of accountability it is necessary to consider separately these two different elements or discourses of accountability.

Munro & Mouritson (1996, p. 3) suggest that the structural perspective on accountability focuses on the measurement of individual performance, issues of target, output and control, establishment of centres of calculation and the creation of visibilities. Roberts (1991, 1996) called this an individualising or hierarchical accountability and associated it with what Habermas calls 'purposive rational action' or 'work' and Foucault's notions of disciplinary power. Roberts (1996) argued that this individualising accountability is maintained by the formal structures of organisations, that it obscures the interdependent nature of organisational life and that it is destructive to 'the self'. This structural or individualising understanding of accountability was a major theme evident in Watson (1995), clearly emerging from the earlier Batey & Lewis and Lewis & Batey understanding, as he acknowledges in his introductory chapter.

Munro & Mouritson (1996, p. 3) associate the second or individual discourse of accountability with the work of psychologists and sociologists who represent accountability as the capacity to give an account, explanation or reason. It was this understanding of accountability that characterised Tilley's (1995) discussion of accounts, accounting and accountability in psychiatric nursing. This sense of duality was also explored in the context of nursing by Ryan (1997, p. 118), who suggested that nurses were like amphibians in that they 'inhabit simultaneously two worlds: the world of artificial organisations and the world of natural persons'.

Roberts (1991, 1996) referred to this second discourse or world of natural persons as socialising accountability, which he associates with what Habermas called 'communicative action' or 'interaction' and the concept of the constitution of the self found in the work of Foucault (1979), Merleau-Ponty (1962) and Mead (1934). Roberts (1996) argues that socialising accountability plays a key role in making the self visible both to self and to others. The self of the child is constructed in being held to account or being called to account by others. For Mead the attitude of others makes the self visible and acts as the mirror in which the self is discovered. Roberts (1996, p. 44) brings these ideas together with the statement that:

> ... the self is discovered only in the process of being called to account by others. Accountability in confronting self with the attitudes of others comes thereby both to address, confirm and shape the self. To be held to account by others has the effect of sharpening and clarifying our sense of self.

These definitions assist to better understand this duality present in Sinclair (1995). However, this quotation from Roberts represents a fundamental mistake made in much of the literature. Accountability is only seen as being held or called to account. This focus is also evident in the work of other authors such as Hoskin & Macve (1986, p. 124), who describe being accountable as 'the state of being liable to answer for one's conduct'. However, this imports a power relationship, a relationship characteristic of a hierarchical context of domination. While this might characterise an individualising or hierarchical accountability it effectively eliminates the possibility of a socialising accountability where accounts might be given freely and thereby facilitate the construction of the self (Starkey & McKinlay, 1998, p. 239). While much of accountability can be seen as an extension of power relationships and therefore as a form of control, a free act of giving an account offers the possibility of something different.

Jacobs & Walker (2000) suggest that it is necessary to reorientate our understanding of accountability by acknowledging that accounts might also be freely given. This draws another distinction between an individualising or structural accountability, where an account is required (and therefore is a form of power or domination), and a socialising or individual accountability, where an account is freely given (and therefore does not represent an explicit power relation).

Jacobs & Walker draw on Foucault's ideas on governmentality and technologies of the self, centrally concepts of self-examination and confession (Foucault, 1980, p. 163), to develop this idea of the socialising or individual accountability. They call it accounting for the self. Just prior to his death Foucault revisited the themes of accountability, examination and the construction of the self, significantly revising and extending his work on these subjects. He suggested that his earlier statements on asylums and prisons focused too heavily on techniques of domination and had tended to represent power and governmentality in an over-simplistic light (Foucault, 1988, p. 19). It is this kind of understanding which has tended to dominate the thinking on accountability.

However, Foucault argued that the technologies of examination and confession enabled people to construct and transform themselves (Bernauer, 1987, p. 53; Foucault, 1985, pp. 63, 70). Therefore the most fundamental distinction between the different discourses of accountability is between an accountability required and an accountability freely given. The first is a technology of domination while the second is about constructing the self. The first raises a series of questions about issues of power and visibility. As a form of disciplinary power structures of accountability have the potential to create new patterns of visibility, make institutional boundaries less opaque and enable the local to become visible to the centre. Therefore questions need to be asked about who, what and how:

> Just who is made visible to whom? Are the patterns of visibility symmetrical or otherwise? Can only the centre observe the local? Or can the local also observe the centre? Equally what emphasis is placed on the forging of a visibility within the system of public administration, as compared to the creation of an external account? (Hopwood, 1984, p. 182)

However, accounting for the self raises different kinds of questions. How do these accounts serve to enable the individual to make sense of their world, including their sense of self in the world (Munro & Mouritson, 1996, p. 6)? How are these accounts developed and how are they linked to practices or technologies such as confession and examination? It is with these questions in mind that I turn to a discussion of the nature of accountability in the organisational and institutional context of the NHS and the clinical governance initiative.

Accountability and reform

In an analysis of public sector reform, particularly changes to healthcare, ideas of accountability seem to be writ large. Humphrey *et al.* (1993) characterise the UK public sector reforms as a change in accountability and accountable management, which was underpinned by shifting concepts and definitions of accountability. In their gospel of managerial reform Osbourne and Gaebler (1992) used the term accountability to mean both financial control and market competition. In their summary of the New Public Management Reforms Ferlie *et al.* (1996) devote an entire chapter to the issue of accountability. They suggest that traditional mechanisms of public sector accountability have been eroded as a consequence of the organisational restructuring, with a corresponding loss in probity (Ferlie *et al.*, 1996, p. 197); in effect a shift from public to managerial accountability. Pollitt & Bouckaert (2000) suggest that rather than a simple shift there is a paradoxical tension between a desire to increase political accountability and a desire to increase managerial accountability.

However, within the UK and other Westminster-influenced systems, NPM reforms have placed pressure on traditional concepts of public accountability. This can be understood as a shift away from what Stewart (1984) called probity, process and policy accountability and what Sinclair called public and administrative accountability, towards managerial accountability, particularly a managerial accountability characterised by financial and budgetary control, performance measurement and audit. This is also driven by a structural discourse on accountability, rather than an individual or socialising one.

Are similar changes also evident in the reforms of the UK NHS? Underlying the Griffiths report (NHS Management Inquiry, 1983) was the desire to clarify lines of accountability by having one identified individual who was accountable for the performance of a given healthcare organisation – the now ubiquitous 'general manager'. This also became reflected in an underlying concept of structural accountability. Once the chief executive is established someone can then account to the Secretary of State who can then account to Parliament. Therefore, within the NHS the Permanent Secretary and the NHS Chief Executive are formally designated as accounting officers and have to report to Parliament for the proper expenditure of public money. They are also required to appear before the Public Accounts Committee and to answer points raised by the Comptroller and Auditor-General. This can be seen as a strengthening of political accountability in that the 'responsible person' or 'accounting officer' is now clearly identified. However, it is also evidently driven by a structural discourse on accountability characterised by the desire to establish visibility, centres of calculation and control.

The various elements of the 1991 reforms to the NHS can also be seen as an effort to restructure accountability. On the demand side the NHS was restructured around the idea of the market with district health authorities (DHAs) and GP fundholders 'purchasing' medical services from the independent 'managerially orientated' NHS trusts. Following Williamson's (1975) argument about markets and hierarchies the introduction of the market would seem to make structures of accountability redundant, as accountability would be understood as a characteristic of an hierarchy rather than a market. Within the NHS trusts the most obvious change was the increased emphasis on managerial accountability. Within the bounds of contracted services issues of efficiency and effectiveness were the responsibility of the trust's general manager. The concept of structural managerial accountability was centrally enshrined in the three objectives established for NHS trusts – they must earn 6% return on assets, they must break even on an annual basis and they must stay within their external financing limits (Bartlett & Le Grand, 1993, p. 54).

The election of a Labour Government in 1997 saw the explicit rejection of the internal market and the purchaser-provider split developed under the Tories and a move towards the use of phrases such as 'integrated care' and quality. The definition of the Labour NHS policy initiatives can be found in the White Paper *The New NHS* (Department of Health, 1997). Central themes of the White Paper were partnership, local delegation, efficiency, integration, technology, the desire to cut administrative costs and improve efficiency, and clinical governance.

While the document was strongly rhetorical it was clear that much of the managerial autonomy of the NHS trusts would be retained. If anything this would be strengthened, with further emphasis on better use of resources, more efficiency and less administration. However, it was also clear that there were to be direct initiatives to increase the use of technology, improve access, shorten waiting lists and that new standards and agencies would be introduced to monitor quality. From a political accountability perspective the relationship for trusts changed in that the trusts would be accountable to the Health Board. Within these changes managerial accountability was strengthened through the increased use of budgetary delegation and performance incentives:

> Efficiency will be enhanced through incentives at both NHS trust and clinical team level. Many NHS trusts already devolve budgetary responsibility to clinical teams and involve senior professionals from them directly in the management of the NHS trust. All NHS trusts should be developing these approaches. (Department of Health, 1997, p. 49)

The recommendation was made that both doctors and nurses would have an increased say in shaping services and that clinical and financial responsibility would be aligned. In England this would involve the delegation of a single unified budget to primary care groups who would have the power to commission and to provide services. However, in Scotland there was not the same financial delegation and commissioning role for the primary care groups.

From an accountability perspective these changes can be seen as an extension and continuation of the previous focus on structural managerial accountability. Although some elements of political accountability, such as the relationship between the NHS trusts and the Health Boards, were clarified or altered, managerial accountability was the key objective. However, there was also a strong emphasis on quality, inspection, evaluation and common standards. Many of these themes came to be grouped together under the heading of clinical governance.

Clinical governance

Within the UK the concept of clinical governance has become associated with issues of quality improvement, clinical audit and corporate governance. However, prior to the Labour NHS policy initiatives the term was not evident in the literature (Walshe, 2000). Within the 1997 White Paper (Department of Health, 1997) clinical governance was defined as:

> A new initiative in this white paper (chapter 6) to assure and improve clinical standards at local levels throughout the NHS. This includes action to ensure that risks are avoided, adverse events are rapidly detected, openly investigated and lessons learned, good practice is rapidly disseminated and systems are in place to ensure continuous improvements in clinical care.
> (Department of Health, 1997, p. 82)

Initially the idea of clinical governance was an extension of earlier models of quality assurance and clinical audit. However, it was also deeply influenced by the experience of the Bristol enquiry into paediatric cardiac surgical deaths and the exposure of the general practitioner Harold Shipman who was found guilty of the unlawful killing of many of his elderly patients. Therefore one central theme has been the problem of 'bad apples' and the identification of adverse events, especially associated with hospitalisation.

The Government developed the clinical governance agenda for England and Wales in the 1998 White Paper *A First Class Service: Quality in the New NHS* (Department of Health, 1998) which was followed in 1999 by a health services circular – *Clinical governance: quality in the new NHS* (Department of Health, 1999a). Davies & Mannion (2000) summarise the main components of clinical governance as:

Clear lines of responsibility and accountability for the overall quality of care. This includes giving the chief executive the ultimate responsibility for clinical quality, and placing an obligation on NHS trusts to arrange formal reporting structures that put quality issues on an even footing with financial matters.

A comprehensive programme of quality improvement activities, such as clinical audit, evidence-based practice, continuing professional development and engagement with national standards are suggested. Clear policies aimed at managing risks involve an emphasis on personal clinical responsibility and the need for systemic reduction of risk. Effective procedures to identify and remedy poor performance include key actions such as critical incident reporting and patient complaint procedures.

The clinical governance agenda as contained in *A First Class Service: Quality in the new NHS* (Department of Health, 1998) and in *Clinical Governance: Quality in the new NHS* (Department of Health, 1999a) had three main ele-ments. The first was the establishment of a set of national quality standards through national service frameworks and the National Institute for Clinical Excellence (NICE). NICE was charged with appraising research evidence on alternative drugs and treatments and producing clear evidence-based guidelines and standards for expected practice.

The second element focused on the clinical governance processes and professional self-regulation at the local level, particularly principles of clinical audit and lifelong learning. The third element was a system for monitoring delivery. Centrally this involved the establishment of a statutory Commission for Health Improvement, an NHS performance assessment framework and a national survey of patient and user experience. Davies & Mannion suggest that this Commission for Health Improvement can be seen as a waiting policeman to deal with miscreants.

From a basic analysis of these documents it becomes evident that the clinical governance initiative is a system of accountability. This is clear in Davies & Mannion's analysis, which starts with the accountability of the chief executive for quality and the responsibility of trusts to measure and report quality. The quality improvement activities emphasise measurement, audit, inspection and comparison to established standards, all of which represent a particular interpretation of the concept of accountability. The idea of account-ability was embedded into the very definition of clinical governance:

A framework through which NHS organisations are accountable for con-tinuously improving the quality of their services and safeguarding high standards of care by creating an environment in which excellence in clin-ical care will flourish.   (Department of Health, 1999a, p. 3)

In Scotland the elements of clinical governance were outlined in two main guidance letters: MEL(1998)75 and MEL(2000c)29. These present a picture similar to the English developments. Trusts have an explicit responsibility for quality and chief executives are accountable for quality performance in the same way as for financial performance. The difference in the Scottish system is that it is more explicitly focused on the trust with less emphasis on external agencies and reviews. NHS trust boards are expected to lead the development of clinical governance, each trust is required to establish a clinical governance committee and trust boards are accountable for quality and the essential monitoring of clinical quality, although there is the provision for national guidelines through the Clinical Standards Board for Scotland. Within MEL(1998)75 there is an interesting and important emphasis on the idea of accountability.

> Clinical governance, as such, is about the 'governance' of the Health Service, and thus about accountability and about structures and processes. . . . Clinical governance is not the sum of all these activities: rather it is the means by which these activities are brought together into a structured framework and linked to the corporate agenda of NHS bodies.

In summary the clinical governance initiative in England and in Scotland can be seen as the establishment of new systems and lines of accountability. Essentially it can be seen as a structural initiative, with the establishment of clear and explicit national goals for quality, institutional obligations to measure and report performance in quality terms, and the creation of inspection and review agencies to ensure that the system operates at a local level. Many existing practices that had ambiguous or multiple lines of accountability, such as professional staff development and clinical audit, were restructured on a structurally-orientated political and managerial tangent.

At a broader level the reform to the UK public sector and more specifically to the NHS can be seen as a shift towards structural models of accountability, particularly a stronger emphasis on clear lines of political accountability and a growing emphasis on concepts of managerial, political and to a lesser extent public accountability. As a consequence issues of professional and personal accountability and the discourse of the individual or accounting for the self have been de-emphasised or conscripted for other ends.

The concept of accountability as contained within the clinical governance framework has been used to emphasise and strengthen the control of politicians not only over financial resources but also over issues previously the primary domain of the professional: quality and performance measurement. In terms of the question of who is accountable to whom it is evident that nurses are now more explicitly accountable to management and through management to the politicians. Using Ryan's (1997) terminology this is about accountability in the world of artificial organisations and for Tilley (1995) this is a third-person 'trace' accountability or reified aspect of a hierarchical social control system rather than the face-to-face accountability of a shared life.

Tilley represents mental illness as a failure to account, and that the role of the nurse is to assist the patient to learn how to do this. Patients can be regarded as persons who interact with nurses because they cannot account for their experience or behaviour (Tilley, 1995, p. 110). Competence in accounting is itself a form of social competence, which may be limited if a person's stock of social knowledge is inadequate (for example if the patient has, through illness or institutionalisation, lost contact with ordinary life, its activities and ways of accounting for it) (Tilley, 1995, p. 111). Accounts are forms of social action that accomplish attribution of or relief from responsibility for social action. Thus they realize – i.e. make real and enable others to grasp – social acts (Tilley, 1995, p. 113).

Within our theoretical framework this can be clearly seen as an example of an individual discourse of accountability. Accounts are not required by a structural hierarchy but are part of establishing and consolidating the self. Tilley's dialogues show these accounts in actions and how the patient is taught to construct and transform him/herself, from the patient into the 'healthy' individual. Also the dialogues show how psychiatric nurses examine and confess their own behaviour, constructing the self of the caring patient-centred nurse.

This idea of an individual discourse of accountability, accounting for the self, is evident in UKCC guidelines. It is also evident, although not so explicit, in the NMC code. The individual discourse is present in the obligation of the nurse to weigh up the interest of clients in situations of conflicting demands and be prepared to account for the decision made (UKCC, 1996a, p. 8). In effect nurses must examine their own behaviour and judgements and confess this, primarily to themselves but potentially to some other individual, be it the patient, colleagues or the UKCC/NMC. It is this act of examination and confession, the process of accounting for the self, which constructs the nurse and makes the difference between those who are and are not nurses. It is this accounting rather than some formal registration process that makes the nurse. This is also at variance with Ryan's claim that it is the patient mandate that makes the nurse.

While a patient may be necessary to practice nursing it is the fact that nurses worry about how they treat their patients and reflect on what they have done that constitutes the difference between a nurse and a non-nurse. A patient will unquestioningly accept the work of someone in a nurse's uniform and in some cases, such as coma patients, theatre or mental healthcare, there may be no patient mandate at all. Yet nurses can still function in these settings. However, it is Ryan's concept of the 'warderly' which emphasises the importance of reflection, examination and accounting in making the nurse. The danger is that the nurse ceases to care, to worry, to reflect, to account to him/herself and examine his/her actions; and in ceasing to care the care ceases.

Perhaps Watson (1992) is right when he suggests that accountability is the essence of professionalism, but this is an individual rather than a structural accountability. If this individual or personal form of accountability is suppressed, excluded or conscripted, then nursing has ceased to exist. Lewis

& Batey's case for structural accountability to the exclusion of other forms is the case for the end of care and the end of nursing.

Conclusion

Upon reflection it is clear that the nursing profession has become confused in its understanding of accountability. Some of the confusion can be traced to Lewis & Batey and their reduction of accountability to a structuralist hierarchy and control. However, this is not a mere definitional problem. Within a context of health reform and managerialist hierarchy the danger is that in embracing hierarchical accountability as an aspect of professionalism nurses could be compromising the very professional status they are seeking to secure, further re-enforcing their subordination to doctors and losing autonomy within the managerial and political hierarchy of the NHS. Abbott (1988) roundly criticises the simple 'characteristic' model of professional development, and argues instead that different groups compete with each other for jurisdiction and status.

In passively accepting power relations involved in structural hierarchy nurses are therefore losing rather than developing their professional status. This is not to suggest that there is a simple correspondence with personal accountability being good and a structural accountability being bad. However, nurses need to understand that accountability is part of a system of control and therefore of power and visibility. Accountability should not be blindly accepted as an example of professional status but seen as a potential zone of conflict and competition between different professional groups and interests.

Returning to Hopwood's (1984) questions about visibility and the concept of accountability, they key question is who is visible to whom. On the whole the reform of the UK public sector has been about making the activities of governmental organisations more visible to the politicians, and therefore about the creation of structures with direct and explicit lines of accountability to the minister. Central elements of this have been an explicit accountability for the use of financial resources and performance. Within the restructured organisations there has also been an explicit effort to create a managerial accountability. These themes have been clearly evident in the reform of the NHS. The chief executive of each trust answers to the Secretary of State and all staff answer to the chief executive. Accountability is the product of location within the healthcare hierarchy and the obligation to answer to a superior for the performance of delegated duties.

The development of the clinical governance initiative can also be seen as part of the attempt to strengthen political and managerial accountability within a structural framework. The central features of this initiative are the desire to create clear lines of accountability, vesting the responsibility for quality in the organisational structure, particularly in the person of the chief executive, and to implement forms of control, measurement, standardisation and inspection operated from the centre.

From the nursing perspective this offers a serious challenge to other concepts and elements of accountability. Within the literature such as Tilley (1995) and the material from the NMC, alternative professional and personal forms of accountability are evident and are articulated within an individual discourse. Accounts are freely given to the self, to the patient and to others as part of the process of being a nurse. In many ways this resolves Watson's (1992) paradox. Accounting to the patient is a form of accountability but it is an individual and sense-making process rather than a form of structural control.

It is important to understand that professional identity is constructed on two levels, externally in terms of claims to professional status, jurisdiction, public trust and state registration (Abbott) and internally in terms of identity, self and accountability. In conclusion perhaps Watson (1992) is quite right when he says that accountability is the essence of professionalism. However, this is an individual professionalism, construction of the self as a nurse rather than some external territorial claim.

The danger evident in the wider process of public sector reform and in the specific changes to the NHS is that the discourse on accountability has been dominated by a structural perspective. Accountability is seen as a process of domination and control and increasingly articulated in the political, public and managerial forms. Within the clinical governance framework concepts of professional and personal accountability are either sidelined or conscripted to a process of political and managerial control. The danger of this is that the element of care and personal reflection present in nursing is suppressed and the nurse is reduced to the functional role of the 'warderly' (Ryan, 1997).

Therefore, it is very important that the value of a discourse of individual accountability in nursing be strongly articulated. Perhaps to maintain this understanding nurses need a mechanism separate from the organisational hierarchy, somewhere or somebody who will facilitate their self-examination and hear their confession and a companion or group who will assist them to balance the conflicting demands and the inherent ambiguity of nursing practice.

Chapter 4
Accountability and Clinical Governance

Roger Watson

Introduction

The purpose of this chapter is to examine the relationship between account-ability and clinical governance. I consider accountability to be a framework for exercising the professional aspects of the work of nurses and midwives: those parts of their roles and jobs for which they have been trained and educated. Nurses and midwives may be called to account formally, either continually as part of the normal course of their work, or periodically, for example, when things go wrong.

I maintain that accountability is the hallmark of a profession (Watson, 1995). My view remains that accountability is a worthy pursuit for nurses and that the periodic exercising of accountability – when things go wrong – is only really possible if nurses learn to be accountable continually. Nurses do account regularly for their activities in nursing records, handing over between shifts, to senior nurses and to medical and other professional colleagues. However, the above accountability is imposed or required by others. Nurses and midwives should be prepared at all times to explain and justify actions in the planning, execution and documentation of care.

If such accountability is the hallmark of professionalism then my question for the purposes of this chapter is 'does clinical governance enhance or detract from the professionalism of nurses and midwives?' If it does detract from it, then does it matter? In addressing this question, a great deal of the evidence I cite comes from medicine. This is because the nursing literature has been largely uncritical of clinical governance or its components and the issues in medicine are mostly directly applicable to nursing and midwifery. Nursing and midwifery may differ from medicine in the extent to which their pro-fessionalism and autonomy are recognised, but what may constitute a threat to professionalism and accountability in medicine surely applies to nursing and midwifery.

Clinical governance

An examination of clinical governance is required before the above questions can be answered. There are various views of what clinical governance is and the concept is viewed from various perspectives in other chapters of this book. Of course, there is a definition of clinical governance:

> A framework through which NHS organisations are accountable for continuously improving the quality of their services and safeguarding high standards of care, by creating an environment in which excellence in clinical care will flourish.   (Department of Health, 1998)

However, like most definitions, it does not provide much meaning. Meaning, as opposed to definition, comes when those who are expected to understand a concept are able to implement it. It gains meaning when they can really explain how it affects them, what they do now that they did not do before and, in the case of nursing and midwifery, how it makes practice and especially patient care, better.

The jury remains out on whether or not clinical governance makes any difference to patient care by nurses (Elcoat & Raymond, 2001) and it is not even clear if everyone has the same understanding of the term. Turnbull (2002) included the term clinical governance in her book *The good and the bad and the gobbledegook: review of tackling NHS jargon*, where it was described as 'technical jargon'. While it may be that a few professionals have a common understanding I have certainly found varying definitions in my own work in an NHS trust. Some claim it is nothing new, just an umbrella term for things that were already in place, while others are more elaborate.

Clinical governance is certainly visible through additional paperwork, structures and committees but the link to better practice or improved care remains to be made. The same could be said, perhaps, of accountability but, assuming that both accountability and clinical governance have their merits, are they just the same thing, two sides of the same coin, or instead antagonistic concepts? In short, are we liable to improve the professionalism of nurses and midwives by continuing to pursue accountability and professionalism or do we need clinical governance in order to achieve this?

Why do we have clinical governance?

Clinical governance is a manifestation of public and Government frustration with the health services generally. In this light it is worth quoting the current UK Chief Medical Officer, Sir Liam Donaldson, from a co-authored article (Halligan & Donaldson, 2001, p. 1413):

> Clinical governance was introduced at the end of a decade in which quality had been more explicitly addressed than ever before. It offers a means to integrate previously rather disparate and fragmented approaches to quality

improvement – but there was another driver for change. The series of high profile failures in standards of NHS care in Britain over the past five years caused deep public and professional concern and threatened to undermine confidence in the NHS. Unwittingly, these events seem to have fulfilled a key criterion for achieving successful change in organisation – the need to establish some urgency.

Everything that anyone could ever want to know about why there is such a thing as clinical governance is encapsulated in the above statement: the reasons, the components and the intentions. The reasons are actually quite hard to grasp: there was a plethora of quality initiatives in the NHS which brought no improvement and, in some cases, failed spectacularly to achieve anything. Medical scandal still exists. Instead of changing tack, the solution has been to leave all the initiatives in place and bring them under one framework. In other words, create and add yet another initiative. The components are all of the extant quality initiatives such as evidence-based practice, clinical audit and so on, and the aims are to improve quality of care in the NHS. In addition, the National Institute for Clinical Excellence (NICE: www.nice.org.uk) was created as well as the Commission for Health Improvement (CHI).

The title of NICE suggests that it has something to do with excellence. However, a closer examination of what NICE was actually established to do shows that it is about reducing 'the likelihood of unacceptable variation in the provision of care epitomised by the availability of expensive drugs in some health authorities and not in others' (Littlejohns, 2001, p. 40). This sounds like a laudable aim, but the easiest way in which to achieve it is to prevent any expensive drugs being available anywhere and there is already some evidence that this has happened with several drugs (Eaton, 2002; Kmietowicz, 2002). The real impingement of NICE, however, is on the clinical judgement of individual doctors.

The other plank of clinical governance, CHI (www.nhs.chi.uk) has the aim of improving the quality of patient care in the NHS. To date, it appears only to have highlighted further examples of poor care across the country and it is not entirely clear how such a body could bring about improvements, far less demonstrate them, when this is the job of individual practitioners. Nevertheless, it is almost heretical to criticise clinical governance: it is well meaning and seeks the best outcomes for patients and, at another level, it gives professionals, such as nurses and midwives and the health service within which they work, guidance on how best to work. However, does it offer anything additional over and above professional accountability? Are there ways in which it could detract from professional accountability and are there other aspects of clinical governance which could be criticised on the basis that they may not lead to better patient care?

Not everyone is convinced about clinical governance. As mentioned above (Elcoat & Raymond, 2001) there are some who think it will not lead to better patient care and an example of how it could lead to worse patient care will be provided below. However, the real issue is the potential damage that clinical governance could do and, in the sphere of medicine, this has been forcefully articulated by James Willis in his book *Friends in Low Places* (2001) where he especially attacks one of the major planks of clinical governance: evidence-based medicine. The problem with evidence-based medicine, according to Willis, is that:

> Doctors are being constrained not to rely on their hard-won experience, knowledge and skill, their <u>unarticulated</u> sense of what needs to be done. But instead always to use their conscious brain function to <u>work out</u> a solution. Thus quite possibly reducing their effectiveness by half.

In fact, the aims of evidence-based practice are described as 'a new paradigm' by one of its supporters (Lockett, 1997, p. 15) who continues to say that it:

> makes explicit the scenario that the clinician is able to critically appraise and use the evidence to provide optimal treatment care. It also places much more of an emphasis on the individual doctor and less on the role of experts.

It is clear, then, that evidence-based medicine is being used to drive forward a departure from previous practice – something which I think its originators never envisaged (Sackett *et al.*, 1997) – and that expertise, honed through experience is now of less importance. There is a naive assumption that experts can be dispensed with and that almost anyone with the most basic level of training and education in medicine can practice like a consultant if they apply the principles of evidence-based medicine. It is unlikely to be this simple.

Of course, there is a fundamental problem of misunderstanding statistics amongst those who promote clinical governance and this is highlighted by Willis. He says that there is a total lack of acceptance that any risk should be tolerated and the fact that half of our doctors are below average performance must be rectified – when, wherever the average lies, half will always be below it. Willis does not eschew the requirement for evidence, of course, but he says 'that evidence-based medicine goes wrong when it stops trying to help, and starts trying to control. In other words, when it stops being a tool, and starts to become a master' (p. 105).

This is essentially the situation we have reached; quality initiatives and frameworks have moved from being tools to draw upon in order for professionals to do their job better and have been elevated to 'master' status within clinical governance. There is certainly accountability within the clinical governance framework but the accountability is imposed, pervasive and institution-centred. Advocates of clinical governance who examine the concept of accountability within it emphasise this last point. For example, McSherry & Pearce (2002, p. 54) see accountability of individuals (and teams and organisations) in terms of 'having the responsibility for implementing, monitoring and evaluating the key components of clinical governance within their role'. It seems that accountability can only exist within a clinical governance framework and they compound this (p. 55) by suggesting, amongst other things, that health professionals who are truly accountable and fit for practice must ensure that their practice is 'evidence-based', 'efficient and effective'. These are clearly institutionally-based criteria for accountability which say little or nothing about the relationship between practitioners and individual patients.

Willis is not alone in the medical field in noting the limits of evidence-based medicine. Professor J. Lobo Antunes in his opening address to the Association for Medical Education in Europe in Lisbon, Portugal, on 29 August 2002 said that, as a result of evidence-based medicine, doctors were becoming 'more concerned with applying findings than with dealing with the patient'. He continued to say that 'evidence-based medicine will not help us to treat the stochastic elements of the human condition: the cantankerous, the recalcitrant or the person who is more interested in alternative approaches'. Medical education 'must teach people what evidence is, about controls and about error and random variation so that they know this when they encounter it in their practice'. Antunes' message is that, instead of providing constraining frameworks for practice, we must educate people properly and leave them to do their job: we must trust them, and the issue of trust will be considered in more depth below.

Poor care

Under what circumstances might clinical governance be in conflict with accountability and lead to poorer patient care? Clinical governance and its components are very target driven, with high targets for throughput and adverse consequences. In the care of older people, falls is one area where the Government (supported by a national service framework (Department of Health, 2001b)) wishes to see a reduction in incidence. Clearly, this is a laudable aim: falls lead to injury and death and if they happen in hospital they lead to longer stays in higher risk environments. However, action around the prevention of falls can lead to reduction in the human rights of older people and it is not clear how these human rights are taken into account within clinical governance.

The easiest way to prevent falls is to prevent the movement of older people. They can be confined to bed, to a chair or simply within a 'safer' environment. In order to achieve this a variety of aids can be used, cot sides being a classic example, and some of these aids lead to greater risk, not necessarily of falling, but of injury from a fall (Watson, 2001). All such restraints have harmful consequences in their own right. If falls in older people are approached from a clinical governance, audit or inspection perspective then there will undoubtedly be overt pressure to reduce falls and there will be covert pressure to reduce falls by any means – including restraint.

In the event that someone falls then a clinical governance framework will record this as an adverse event. Clearly, explanations may be required in order to investigate the fall but there will be pressure not to let this happen again. An older person may have fallen because it was judged not to be in their best interests that they be restrained. The interaction between clinical governance and professional accountability was noted by Ballinger & Payne (2002, p. 319) in a study of falls in older people. They said that it:

> appears that the increasing focus on the health professionals' responsibility to maintain the safety of service users, partly through the rigid interpretation of professional rules of conduct, may also contribute to a conservative approach to service provision in which patient-initiated activity is seen as potentially challenging and dangerous.

Within a framework where professional accountability is prevalent, rather than governance, the nurses involved are encouraged to be accountable both in care planning and, if a fall takes place, for the care they have delivered. An accountability framework leaves more room for people to give accounts and to think in accountable terms. In the meantime, older people may suffer the multiple adverse effects of immobility (Watson, 2001).

Short cuts

Another criticism of clinical governance is that it is meant to be a short cut. Like most short cuts, it is designed to reach a particular destination faster but to miss out a great deal in the process. Short cuts are liable to leave those who took them wishing that they had taken the longer route for want of the experience they might have gained along the way (Watson, 2002) and experience is a crucial part of professional development. Moreover, short cuts often take longer – they only look short. All this supports Willis' point presented earlier about reducing the effectiveness of doctors by insisting that they follow the evidence-based medicine route rather than relying on experience and judgement.

It is the short-cutting aspects of governance which put it most at odds with professional accountability. Clearly, some order must be brought to the potential chaos of a health service – there must be some way to predict the likely profile of patients passing through the service and there must be some way in which standards can be set within a quality framework in order to gauge if the service is being successful or not. However, governance views success from a global and collective perspective. This is very sensitive to Government policy, to the prevailing economic climate and to the latest whims of pressure and special interest groups. This is completely at odds with individual patient care.

Professional and individual accountability is the only way in which individualised care can be met that is actually in the best interests of the patient. Such care may well operate within particular financial constraints – the health services cannot meet the bottomless pit of demand – but if nurses and midwives know that what drives their work is their individual accountability for their actions with each patient then they are more likely to act in the best interests of that patient rather than meet predetermined targets which may be at odds with those interests. Referring to the example of falls in older people, nurses who are exercising personal and professional accountability are more likely to permit older people to take risks in line with their personal wishes and dignity if they are permitted to give an account at the end of the day for their actions.

Trust

The final issue to be considered is trust. In relation to Antunes' lecture above I contrasted control via the use of evidence-based medicine, one of the main planks of clinical governance, with trusting appropriately trained and accountable professionals to get on with their jobs. The issue of trust was the subject of the Reith Lectures *A question of trust* sponsored by the British Broadcasting Corporation in 2002 and delivered by Onora O'Neill, Principal of Newnham College, Cambridge (O'Neill, 2002). O'Neill asks if the concept of trust is failing and claims that there is evidence that we trust less than we used to. At least, we say that we trust less than we do, when we are asked about it, despite the fact that we still obviously use the professions frequently.

However, this reporting of a lack of trust has been picked up and seized by our political masters and used as a rod to beat us with, in search of what O'Neill describes as a 'more perfect accountability'. The outcome of this search for better accountability 'lies in prevention and sanctions . . . institutions and professionals should be made more accountable'. In the public sector the new accountability takes the form of 'detailed control' articulated in an 'unending stream of new legislation and regulation'. Without being specific about it, clinical governance fits this particular bill perfectly and the work of health trusts is included. Quoting liberally from O'Neill:

> The new legislation, regulation and controls are more than fine rhetoric. They required detailed conformity to procedures and protocols, detailed record keeping and provision of information in specified formats and success in reaching targets. Detailed instructions regulate and prescribe the work and performances of health trusts and schools, of universities and research councils, of the police force and of social workers.

Ignoring the mass of regulations and frameworks is out of the question as 'the new accountability has quite sharp teeth'. But the most disturbing aspect of the new accountability and the most relevant to this chapter is that:

> The new accountability is widely experienced not just as changing but I think as distorting the proper aims of professional practice and indeed as damaging professional pride and integrity. Much professional practice used

to centre on interaction with those whom the professionals serve: patients and pupils, students and families in need.

Under the system of new accountability professionals are all too busy conforming to the tenets of the creed to fulfil their professional duty. O'Neill describes this as compiling evidence 'to protect themselves against the possibility not only of plausible, but of far-fetched complaints'.

Conclusion

This chapter has tried to assess accountability in the light of clinical governance. The former has been described as the hallmark of professionalism while the introduction of clinical governance can be viewed as a threat to professionalism and that threat comes about through the redirection of accountability away from the individual being accountable for their practice towards the individual being accountable within a predetermined framework. The difference lies in the reduced ability of professionals to account for practice which they deem appropriate on the basis of their education, training and experience – which they consider to be in the best interests of their patients – within an accountability framework where the targets are predetermined and restrictive. An example was provided of how action to reduce falls in older people, if approached from a clinical governance perspective, could lead to worse care despite a reduction in falls.

The chapter has not focused purely on nursing and midwifery. Examples from medicine have been used because professional accountability is common to nursing, midwifery and medicine and there has been more evidence of the effects of clinical governance on medicine. On the whole, nursing appears acquiescent to the new paradigm of governance frameworks and in many NHS trusts nurses take the lead in clinical governance.

As this chapter was being written the leader of the British Medical Association, Ian Bogle (2002), quoted in the *Daily Telegraph*, came out clearly against the 'tick-box' mentality which had become prevalent in the 'tick-box NHS'. The 'tick-box' mentality refers to the need to satisfy managerial requests for information, as required under clinical governance, without any indication that there is any improvement in patient care. In fact, Bogle maintains that there is no improvement in patient care and his view is consistent with others who have been cited above such as Willis and Antunes. In a telling statement Bogle, no longer in practice, says:

> By the time I left, my practice was restricted by prescribing guidelines, referral guidelines and the threat of litigation if I chose, on occasion, to trust my judgement, take a risk and act outside accepted protocols for the treatment of certain conditions.

He reckoned that he was unable 'to get patients the care and treatment (he) knew they needed . . . clinical decisions have been taken out of clinicians' hands'.

The phenomenon of the new accountability, as it is described by O'Neill in her 2002 Reith lectures, extends beyond medicine, nursing and social work. For example, it is prevalent in education at primary, secondary and tertiary levels. In this respect nursing suffers from a 'double whammy' effect whereby it is scrutinised in practice and also in the process of nursing education. Again, the 'tick-box' mentality has been equally criticised in education by a former headmaster of a religious public school in England who reckoned that education was being taken over by a culture of 'box-ticking bureaucrats' who viewed education as a 'box-ticking exercise' which was wearing down teachers (Thompson & Clare, 2002, quoted in the *Daily Telegraph*). The process was likened to trying to fatten a pig simply by weighing it: everything had to be measured but what was it that the UK Government was actually measuring?

With reference to this book, which is really concerned with the notions of accountability and clinical governance in nursing and midwifery, what relevance does anything from medicine or education have? A great deal, in my opinion. Education and medicine are robust professions with long histories and the erosion of professionalism, through reduction of the ability to exercise personal accountability, has been rapid and effective. Nursing continues to strive for professional status and remains ambivalent about the place of personal and professional accountability in its practice. Midwifery has gained autonomy to a greater extent but how much more vulnerable is nursing than medicine? Again, a great deal in my opinion and the likelihood of accountability being recognised as a worthy pursuit for nurses and midwives must be at risk within a clinical governance framework.

However, clinical governance is unlikely to go away, trust in professions has been eroded and control has been taken from them. Control is usually removed and rarely restored and, while the prospect of better patient care within a clinical governance framework may seem unlikely, the challenge for nurses and midwives remains: to tick the boxes that require to be ticked but not to lose sight of the real focus, the individual who requires us.

Chapter 5

The Legal Accountability of the Nurse

John Tingle

Introduction

The broad aim of this chapter is to analyse the legal accountability of the nurse according to the law of negligence, taking into account the current clinical negligence healthcare environment.

The concept of accountability and the new NHS

In the past decade or so there have been changes in the law and more markedly in Government policy towards the rights of patients and their relationship with healthcarers. Under *The NHS Plan* (Department of Health, 2002b) the patient is meant to be king in the new NHS. The concept of 'Patient Empowerment' is the directing Government policy imperative (Tingle, 2002) which can be seen to permeate the development of health and through to the new health quality institutions in the NHS: organisations such as CHI (Commission for Health Improvement), NICE (National Institute for Clinical Excellence) and NPSA (National Patient Safety Agency) to name but a few. These, and a number of other organisations, have been created by the Government to advance the quality of patient care (Tingle, 2002).

The patient is now to be seen by healthcarers and all those concerned with the NHS as the most important person in the NHS and this policy imperative has clear implications for the concept of accountability. The conventional wisdom seems to be, certainly in Government health quality policy making and increasingly at the grass-roots level of healthcare delivery, that accountability to the patient is now implicit in the care relationship. It could be argued that today, it almost goes without saying that the healthcarer is accountable to the patient. In the last decade the UKCC was trying hard to push the idea of accountability and patient advocacy, which was commendable and far-sighted of them. The concrete has now set in respect of the accountability concept and other ideas such as patient empowerment, clinical governance, transparency of function and clinical risk management, to name but a few concepts currently in vogue.

The Human Rights Act 1998 is also in force now and it maintains an important rights focus. The Act has important implications for all healthcarers (Garwood Gowers *et al.*, 2001). Patients have used the Act for a variety of reasons in a variety of clinical areas, successfully recently in *Regina (Rose and Another) v. Secretary of State for Health and Another, The Times,* 22 August 2002, where children born by artificial insemination claimed access to certain non-identifying information relating to their donors which facilitated the establishment of their personal identity. The Human Rights Act 1998 can be regarded as an effective mechanism or tool of securing healthcarer accountability to patients.

Accountability is not irrelevant

The concept of accountability, however, must not be seen as an irrelevance in the new NHS of the Labour Government. It is still a useful label or handle to justify conduct but it must now be seen to exist along with lots of other labels. It is also not as fashionable a concept as it once was and is now, arguably, an accepted part of the patient care equation.

Labels can obscure meanings

The word accountability, as a label, has a number of meanings or senses, which will be explored in this chapter and elsewhere in the book. It is a handy label to describe a complex set of affairs. The important point about labels is that they sometimes can obscure meanings. Understanding and defining a concept such as accountability can eventually become an almost tautological exercise. The nature of academic work is to avoid falling into the tautological trap and to provide signposts and to navigate the reader through the issues and this is the principal objective of works like this and the purpose of this chapter.

Ideas behind the label

Sometimes it is better to look at the ideas behind the label rather than at the label itself. To understand accountability today, the whole structure of the NHS needs to be considered and all the health quality improvement organisations contained within it, as patient accountability is the concept which underpins and is behind them all. This is an impossibly tall order but is reflective of the reality that exists. Accountability can now be seen to have gone 'live' in today's NHS.

This chapter

This chapter is largely unchanged from the original as the law and the commentary are still applicable. Due to limitations of space, however, the topic of health resources and the law has been consolidated. A more detailed treatment is given elsewhere (Garwood Gowers *et al.*, 2001, Stauch *et al.*, 2002).

Legal accountability

The law affects everybody and it cannot be ignored. Legal accountability is the prime form of accountability for every citizen, and nurses, like all other professionals, are personally accountable through the law for their actions or omissions. This individual legal accountability is channelled through the criminal and civil law and the courts.

The law maintains an important presumption: that ignorance of it will not excuse should legal action result. Therefore, as a matter of practical necessity nurses, like all other professionals, need to be aware of the legal aspects of their role. The nurse's legal accountability also needs to be contrasted with the other forms of accountability that exist – and these can conflict with each other. It is also possible to view some as being more important than others.

Interests, rights and duties: the role of the law

The law performs a number of general functions in society. It articulates interests, rights and duties and chooses between them when they conflict. Reported cases in health law show this process happening all the time and there can be many interests at stake. Sometimes the cases involve choices between life and death. Cases can involve the State, other individuals, healthcarers and the patient. There are a myriad number of issues that can be seen in the cases that come before the courts, ranging from abortion rights, rights and duties of children and parents regarding consent, refusal of treatment, rights of patients to refuse life-saving treatment amongst others. These cases are decided in courts of law and the law can clearly be seen to be articulating rights and duties and resolving conflicts of interests.

The Ms B. case

The recent Ms B. case is a particularly good example of a court dealing with a very difficult life and death decision and articulating rights and duties. The case, *Ms B. v. an NHS Hospital Trust* [2002] EWHC (Fam) 429, was widely reported in the press. Ms B. was very ill and she did not wish to be kept artificially alive by the use of a ventilator. Dame Elizabeth Butler-Sloss, the President of the Family Division in the High Court of Justice, in deciding that Ms B. could refuse life-saving treatment made reference in her judgment to principles of autonomy, the sanctity of life, and assessing capacity. She stated in her judgment:

> One must allow for those as severely disabled as Ms B., for some of whom life in that condition may be worse than death. It is a question of values

and, as Dr Sensky and Dr Atkins have pointed out, we have to try inadequately to put ourselves into the position of the gravely disabled person and respect the subjective character of experience. Unless the gravity of the illness has affected the patient's capacity, a seriously disabled patient has the same rights as the fit person to respect for personal autonomy. There is serious danger, exemplified in this case, of a benevolent paternalism which does not embrace recognition of the personal autonomy of the severely disabled patient.

This quote mentions values, autonomy and paternalism, which are all key ethical concepts and the judge here can be seen to be balancing these and coming to a reasoned decision. It is difficult to imagine embarking on a more difficult and important legal task.

Dispute resolution, compensation and punishment

The law is also used to resolve disputes, for example, where a patient may have been injured by a nurse and sues for compensation. A practice nurse, for example, may have syringed an ear negligently (Parker & Wilson, 1992) and caused the patient injury. The nurse may deny negligence, and if the case is not settled beforehand the dispute will be resolved in court.

Establishing nursing negligence

The important issues to be determined in this case will be, first, whether the practice nurse owed a legal duty of care to the patient. Broadly speaking, a legal duty of care is owed to our neighbours, people to whom we are proximate and whom we can reasonably foresee will be injured by our actions or omissions. In the doctor-nurse-patient relationship this first element will nearly always be established as it is here, as there is a sufficiently close, proximate relationship.

Second, breach of the legal duty to care has to be established and the basic premise of the reasonable practice nurse would probably be used in the example in order to assess the appropriate legal standard of care to be exercised. The court would seek to find out whether the nurse acted as an ordinary skilled practice nurse would have acted in the circumstances of the case. Expert nurse evidence would be given on this point and the court might look for the exercise of a medical standard of care in the circumstances (Tingle, 2001a).

Regard would also be had as to the conduct of the delegating GP: in other words, whether there was any evidence of wrongful delegation (General Medical Council, 2001). If unreasonable, negligent conduct is established, the person making the claim will then have to establish the third element, i.e. that the injuries received were caused, or materially contributed to by, the negligent conduct of the practice nurse and doctor (who would be the defendants). The harm must also have been reasonably foreseeable, and if all this is established and negligence is found then monetary compensation in the form of damages will be awarded.

Vicarious liability

The GP employer of the practice nurse in the example given will also be liable for the negligence under the principle of vicarious liability. This principle operates to make an employer liable, along with the employee, for any negligence caused by the employee. The negligent practice nurse, however, still remains personally legally liable for any wrongs and could still be sued personally by the injured patient though this would be unlikely. Practice nurses would be unlikely to have the financial resources available to be worth suing personally. However they may have a professional negligence indemnity insurance policy from their trade union or medical defence organisation and this would be a relevant factor to consider. The Nursing & Midwifery Council (NMC, 2002a) considered making it a compulsory requirement for nurses, midwives and health visitors to have indemnity insurance but decided against doing this.

The aim of the law: compensation

The aim of the law in personal injury court actions, where a breach of duty has been proved, is to try and compensate the physically injured claimant (the patient in the above example) as fully as money possibly can for the injuries received, i.e. to put the claimant in the position they would have been in had the wrong not been committed. It is very difficult to put into monetary terms the value of a lost sense or faculty, but nevertheless an attempt is made. In criminal law the focus of the law is different because of the fundamental nature of what has occurred. The convicted person is seen as having committed a crime against society, and therefore society punishes. In civil law the defendant is viewed as having committed a wrong against an individual; therefore civil law is largely concerned with compensation.

Clinical negligence law today: all change?

Clinical negligence litigation is now high on the public agenda. The Government stated in the NHS Plan that it would look to make further changes to the way the NHS handles and responds to clinical negligence claims. Claims' costs are rising and costs can exceed damages for lower value claims.

The National Audit Office (NAO, 2001) states the following key facts on clinical negligence:

- Around 10 000 new claims were received in 1999–2000.
- At 31 March 2000, provisions to meet likely settlements for up to 23 000 outstanding claims were £2.6 billion. In addition, it was estimated that a further £1.6 billion would be required to meet likely settlements for claims

expected to arise from incidents that have occurred but not been reported.
- Only 24% of claims funded by the Legal Services Commission are successful.
- The total annual charge to NHS income and expenditure accounts for provisions for settling claims has risen seven-fold since 1995–96.

These facts are a cause of concern for patients, the Government and all those who work in and with the NHS. If we improve the quality of health-care then claims should be reduced. The Government has been attempting to instill good quality healthcare practices in the NHS by a whole raft of initiatives, which were mentioned above. They are also looking critically at the clinical negligence system itself and have issued a consultation paper on issues and reform and a Government White Paper is promised (Department of Health, 2001a, 2003).

The concept of patient accountability can be seen to be present in the consultation document. The consultation paper states:

> There are clear and common themes emerging through the great mass of public commentary on clinical negligence, which complement much of that regarding perceived weaknesses in the NHS complaints procedure, which we intend to reform as well. We need to develop:
>
> - a more responsive and patient focused approach to both complaints and clinical negligence claims handling, which provides remedies more closely tailored to individual patient's needs – including practical, non-financial and financial remedies which address concerns directly and quickly.
> - greater openness in the NHS to concerns – so patients know they will be heard, and organisations can learn from mistakes – and links with other structures.
> - ways of addressing the spiralling cost of clinical negligence claims and the time it takes to resolve them.   (Department of Health, 2001a)

Reform of the complaints system and the clinical negligence system seems inevitable; the issue is the precise extent of the reform (Tingle, 2001b).

Regulation, deterrence and education: the role of the law

The law has other general functions, such as deterrence, regulation and education.

The deterrent function

This operates when professionals see what happens to others who are negligent or commit crimes. They do not wish to be in the same unenviable position and will reflect on their professional practice and alter it if necessary.

The regulation function
This operates to check professional and public bodies like the NMC and the General Medical Council. The public body may be exercising its powers unlawfully and its actions could be challenged in a court and declared illegal.

The education function
This operates when court cases are reported in the professional nursing and legal literature, whereby more people become aware of the issues and will reflect on their professional practice and alter it if necessary. This education function can usefully be illustrated by the case of *Crawford v. Board of Governors of Charing Cross Hospital*, reported in *The Times* of 8 December 1953 (Tingle & Foster, 2002). The plaintiff, Mr Robert Joseph Crawford, was admitted to hospital for an operation to remove his bladder. The operation involved a blood transfusion and his arm was extended at an angle of 80° from his body so that he could be given the transfusion. He suffered a loss of power in his arm, was later found to be suffering from brachial palsy, and sued for negligence.

The judge in the lower court based his finding of negligence on the anaesthetist's failure to read an article in the *Lancet*, which warned of the danger of brachial palsy in these circumstances. The Court of Appeal allowed the appeal and found no negligence. Lord Denning stated that it would be putting too high a burden on a person to say that they must read every article in the medical press, although there could be a case of negligence where a recommendation becomes so well proven, accepted and known that it should have been read.

If a contributor makes a point in a journal it could be negligence to just rush in and adopt the findings, and much depends on how widely accepted and regarded the research or article is. Mason & McCall-Smith (1994) analyse Crawford and its current implications stating:

> Failure to read a single article, it was said, may be excusable, while disregard of a series of warnings in the medical press could well be evidence of negligence. In view of the rapid progress currently being made in many areas of medicine, and in view of the amount of information confronting the average doctor, it is unreasonable to expect a doctor to be aware of every development in his field. At the same time, he must be reasonably up to date and must know of major developments.

It is an essential element of the professional and legal accountability of nurses that they keep reasonably up to date in their field of practice. A more recent case is *Gascoine v. Ian Sheridan and Co. and Latham* [1994] Med LR 437. This case involved a number of issues, one of which was the responsibility of a hospital consultant to keep informed about changes and developments in his speciality. Mr Justice Mitchell said that the consultant in question was a very busy man:

who clearly had a responsibility to keep himself generally informed on mainstream changes in diagnosis, treatment and practice through the mainstream literature such as the leading textbooks and the *Journal of Obstetrics and Gynaecology*. Equally clearly it would be unreasonable to suppose that [he] had the opportunity to acquaint himself with the content of the more obscure journals.

This case is authority for the proposition that all professionals should be able to demonstrate a personal, systematic and professional updating regime. If nurses argue that they have not got the time to read the main journal or journals of their speciality or fail to attend update courses and just switch off, they are in a vulnerable position. If something untoward happened to a patient that they were treating and it is subsequently found that this incident could have been avoided if they had kept up to date, then they will be open to criticism. Much however will depend on the circumstances of the case.

Evidence-based healthcare and the courts

Allied to the professional updating issues discussed above is the court's current approach to assessing expert nursing and medical evidence in a clinical negligence case. Judges and lawyers are not, generally speaking, qualified in medical and nursing matters and they have to rely on the evidence of experts. An experienced nurse or doctor will give evidence in the case to say what they would have expected the reasonable nurse or doctor to have done in the circumstances and this helps the judge set the appropriate standard of care that should have been exercised.

This approach is much more evidence-based and less deferential than it used to be. Experts' opinions must have a logical basis. Experts must have also directed their minds to the question of comparative risks and benefits and must have reached a defensible conclusion on the matter. This more judicially testing approach to expert evidence fits in well with the concept of clinical governance and what the Government is trying to do in their healthcare reforms. The case which set the baseline for this new approach is *Bolitho v. City and Hackney Health Authority* [1998] Lloyd's Rep Med 26.

The scandals of recent years

The widely reported medical scandals of recent years, e.g. Bristol and Shipman to name but two, have also affected the way medicine and healthcare generally is perceived by the public and to an extent the judiciary (Bristol Royal Infirmary Inquiry, 2001; Shipman Inquiry Reports, 2002–2003). Public deference towards doctors is not as great as it once was. Lord Woolf in *The Times*, 17 January 2001 stated the new judicial conventional wisdom on doctors:

until recently the courts treated the medical profession with excessive deference, but recently the position has changed ... the over deferential
approach is captured by the phrase: 'doctor knows best'. The contemporary approach is a more critical approach. It could be said that doctor knows
best if he acts reasonably and logically and gets his facts right.

Today the courts are more proactive and testing when they are dealing with
a clinical negligence case. The courts can be seen now more strongly to advance
the notion of patient healthcare to the court and the public. The courts
can be seen to be acting as a strong channel and mechanism of healthcarer
accountability.

The law affects all aspects of nursing

The law affects all aspects of nursing practice, from making a cup of tea to
giving injections. In the case of *Pargeter v. Kensington and Chelsea and West-
minster Health Authority*, reported in the *Lancet* of 10 November 1979, a
patient was given a cup of tea the day after having an operation to remove
a cataract. He drank the tea, vomited immediately and his left eye burst open.
Despite further corrective operations he eventually lost the sight in that eye.
The patient sued for damages but was unsuccessful because negligence could
not be established. A number of issues were discussed in the case, including
the practice of testing the patient's tolerance to liquids by giving trial sips.
The judge felt that in this case it was highly improbable that the common
surgical nursing practice of giving trial sips of liquid had not been followed.

In the case of *Smith v. Brighton and Lewes Hospital Management Committee*, reported in *The Times Law Report* of 1 May 1958, the plaintiff received
injuries when a course of streptomycin injections overran. The nursing sister
was found to be negligent in not taking elementary precautions to stop this,
and damages were awarded. She could have drawn a red line or a star on the
treatment sheet to indicate the time when the prescription was to end. Since
she did not do this extra doses were accidentally given by two other nurses.

A number of the functions of law have been identified, discussed and
related to aspects of nursing practice. This process will be continued later
in the chapter, when the nurse's role in healthcare resource allocation and
management is discussed, along with how the courts have become involved
in these issues. However, it is first important in a book which looks at
the various forms of accountability, to explore further the nature of legal
accountability and, specifically, to try and distinguish the nurse's legal
accountability from other types of accountability.

The various forms of accountability

There is no universally agreed definition of the term accountability or a
classification of types (Tingle, 1990). Some definitions have been attempted.
Tschudin (1992) stated:

Accountability means not only having to answer for an action when something goes wrong, but it is a continuous process of monitoring how a nurse performs professionally. The responsibility differs in different situations, but there is a need to be aware that one is constantly responsible, and therefore constantly accountable. A distinction needs to be made between legal and moral accountability.

Lewis & Batey (1982) and Batey & Lewis (1982) stated:

> We define accountability . . . as the fulfillment of a formal obligation to disclose to referent others the purposes, principles, procedures, relationships, results, income, and expenditures for which one has authority.

These definitions are useful starting points or templates from which to conduct an analysis of the concept of accountability. Defining accountability does seem to be tautological – the concept is a broad one, which is, arguably, indefinable. Nevertheless, the exercise of trying is valuable. Thinking at an abstract level does seem to lead to more reflective professional practice: more thought is given to how a job is performed and the personal accountability attached to that job. An understanding of the concept of accountability can arguably be obtained from an individual's common experiences and general perceptions. All nurses should be able to offer a meaningful 'gut reaction' definition of the concept, and of many others such as responsibility, autonomy, justice, fairness and quality of life. The essential flavour would seem to be that of answerability, i.e. giving a reasoned account for one's own actions or omissions.

Accountable to whom?

Having discussed definitions of accountability it is necessary to deal with the issue of the direction of accountability: to who are nurses accountable? Accountability is a multifaceted concept. Arguably, a nurse could be accountable to:

- the profession
- colleagues
- the patient
- the employer
- society
- a professional regulatory body
- the law
- their immediate family
- themselves

These levels of accountability are not all of equal importance: some are more important than others and conflict between them is certainly possible. A nurse may be asked to work on a ward which is chronically understaffed, but does not say anything about the poor working conditions. As a result of the workload, and doing his/her best to cope, the nurse injures a patient in the course of administering an intravenous infusion, which a busy doctor had requested and which he/she was not qualified to do. The nurse knew that he/she lacked the competence to carry out the procedure but wanted to appear helpful and had no time to discuss the matter. All the forms of account-ability can apply here:

- Patient accountability: reading the *Code of Professional Conduct* (NMC, 2002b), the NMC would say that the nurse was primarily accountable to the patient.

- Employer accountability: the nurse's employer would say that the nurse is accountable to them as an employee, by virtue of their contract of employment.

- NMC accountability: the NMC could view their conduct as being pro-fessional misconduct, and disciplinary proceedings could result.

- Society accountability: society has an interest in the situation, as safe hos-pitals are clearly in the public interest and furthermore public money from taxes funds the NHS.

- Legal accountability: the nurse owes a personal legal duty of care to the injured patient. The patient could take legal action for compensation for breach of this legal duty. A judge would hear the evidence and the nurse would have to account for both actions and omissions.

- Self-accountability: the negligent nurse also has to live with the decision taken. They have to answer to themselves and, if possible, justify the misconduct.

- Professional accountability: other nurses would seek explanations of this nurse's conduct. There is a duty not to bring the profession into disrepute.

- Colleague accountability: colleagues would also require an explanation.

- Immediate family accountability: the nurse's immediate family would also be concerned if they were distressed, and would naturally require an explanation.

- Also, as members of the public, taxpayers and users of the NHS, the imme-diate family of the patient has a legitimate right to ask questions.

Accountability and sanctions

In order to understand the different forms of accountability fully it is neces-sary to determine the relative weight of each one. Which form of account-ability can impose the harshest sanction on the nurse for transgression? What is harsh will necessarily be a value judgement, on which there will be dif-ferences of opinion. Logically, harshness can be looked at in terms of the financial and emotional hardship imposed by the accountability body:

- the NMC can remove the nurse from the register
- society, colleagues and family can admonish the nurse
- the employer can dismiss the nurse
- the nurse can hate themselves
- the law can punish the nurse by imprisonment or fine, and can award compensation and the costs of the action

Imprisonment would be the harshest of the sanctions discussed in terms of the emotional and financial hardship imposed. The law is therefore the accountability mechanism that could impose the harshest sanction, and is therefore the one that would have the most direct effect on the nurse.

The allocation and management of healthcare resources: the nurse's role

The NHS has limited resources to meet a seemingly infinite demand for its services. It is, therefore, an inevitable fact of professional life that decisions have to be made on how best to use these resources (Klein & Redmayne, 1992). In the context of the NHS, resource issues do generate a lot of publicity and emotive debate. This is understandable, as the issues at stake are health and, sometimes, life itself: 'Sick boy seeks court ruling on closure' *The Times* of 9 June 1993; and 'Kidney patients die as costly machines lie idle' in *The Times* of 26 July 1993; and *R. v. Cambridge District Health Authority ex parte B* [1995] 2 All ER 129.

Today the NHS has more resources. The Government has an express policy of ending unreasonable regional variations of care. There are national service frameworks, national clinical guidelines and we have NICE. The NHS could still do with more resources but in fairness the Government seems to have made strong efforts today to improve the NHS resource situation. Having said that, on a micro level, in the author's experience, nurses still complain about poor and sometimes dangerous staffing levels.

A conflict of accountability

Nurses can experience a conflict of accountability in this area (Lee, 1995). For example, a hospital manager may feel that the staffing level on one ward is just about safe and therefore acceptable. No other staff can be obtained because of budget restraints. The manager would like more staff but cannot obtain the necessary extra funding. The nurses on duty are aware of the budget problems but feel that poor staffing levels are compromising patient safety. They are employees, who have legal obligations to and are therefore accountable to their employer. They are under a legal duty to cooperate with their employer and to obey all reasonable instructions. Employees must also exercise reasonable care and skill in doing their job. The nurses make their views known to management, but management does nothing about it and tells them to carry on as best they can. The staffing levels remain the same.

What action should follow and how is it linked to the concept of accountability? The nurses are also accountable, as stated above, to the NMC and must ensure that they follow their advice in this situation. The code (NMC, 2002b) in Clause 8 contains key provisions, which can be related to resources:

8.1 You must work with other members of the team to promote healthcare environments that are conducive to safe, therapeutic and ethical practice.

8.3 Where you cannot remedy circumstances in the environment of care that could jeopardize standards of practice, you must report them to a senior person with sufficient authority to manage them and also, in the case of midwifery, to the supervisor of midwives. This must be supported by a written record.

8.4 When working as a manager, you have a duty towards patients and clients, colleagues, the wider community and the organisations in which you and your colleagues work. When facing professional dilemmas, your first consideration in all activities must be the interests and safety of patients and clients.

This common-sense advice is helpful and as can be seen from Clause 8:4 managers are specifically targeted.

The role of the law: legal accountability

In discussing the problem above there is also the legal accountability of the various parties to consider. The nurses, managers, the employing health organisation, all owe the patient a legal duty of care. All the other mechanisms of accountability discussed earlier will apply. If a patient on the ward suffers an injury which could easily have been avoided had there been adequate and proper staffing levels, then there may be a real possibility of legal action and legal accountability will have the most direct effect on all the parties involved in the case. It will be recalled that this legal duty is a duty not to expose the patient to unreasonable risks. It requires people to behave reasonably towards their neighbour. A fundamental question will be the extent to which they all did behave reasonably in the circumstances of the case in question. The nurses, manager and employer could all find themselves in court having to explain themselves. In some circumstances, employers could be directly and not vicariously liable to the injured claimant (Tingle, 2001c).

Cases of resources and negligence

A number of cases of healthcare resources and negligence have gone to court and some of these will be discussed within the context of negligence law. An organisation can be negligent if it does not organise its services properly. As Jones (2002) argues:

> As a general rule a defendant's lack of resources will not justify a failure to take the precautions demanded by the exercise of reasonable care. . . . Impecuniosity is not a defence. It may be relevant, however, where the claimant seeks to hold a public authority liable in negligence for failing to provide an adequate service.

The following cases of negligent organisation of services explore this point.

Bull v. Devon Area Health Authority (1989), [1993] 4 Med LR 117. Mrs Bull went into hospital in premature labour, carrying uniovular twins sharing the same placenta. At 7.27 PM the first twin, later named Darryl, was spontaneously delivered and was a male, class A. The second twin, later named Stuart, was delivered 68 minutes later but was subsequently found to have been born with severe brain damage. Stuart should have been delivered as soon as practicable after the first twin and, in any event, within 20 minutes. Specialist medical staff should have attended Mrs Bull in sufficient time to deal with the sort of emergency that arose in the case. Proper assistance was not readily available and the maternity service was found to be negligently organised. Lord Justice Slade stated: 'In cases where multiple births were involved, the system in operation at the hospital . . . was obviously operating on a knife-edge. It had to be operated with maximum efficiency.'

This judge was prepared to presume negligence from the facts of the case under a legal principle known as *res ipsa loquitur*. The defendants could not satisfactorily explain the delay in securing specialist medical staff. Another senior judge, Lord Justice Dillon, stated:

> The Exeter City Hospital provides a maternity service for expectant mothers, and any hospital, which provides such a service, ought to be able to cope with the not particularly out of the way case of a healthy young mother in somewhat premature labour with twins.

He went on to say that there should have been 'a staff reasonably sufficient for the foreseeable requirements of the patient'.

Lord Justice Mustill addressed the hypothetical argument that the hospital providing a public service had done the best it could with the limited resources it had at its disposal:

> Again, I have some reservations about this contention, which are not allayed by the submission that hospital medicine is a public service. So it is, but there are other public services in respect of which it is not necessarily an answer to allegations of unsafety that there were insufficient resources to enable the administrators to do everything which they would like to do.

The Bull case shows that the courts are not afraid to grapple with the issue of healthcare resources where failure to organise them properly results in negligence. In this case Lord Justice Mustill was not prepared to give the health authority a discount in safety standards because it was a publicly funded NHS hospital.

Another case, which also looks at allegations of negligence and healthcare resources and organisation is in the context of standards of care for the mentally ill in hospital. *Knight and Others v. Home Office and Another* [1990] 3 All ER 237.

Paul Barrington Worrell, aged 21 years, committed suicide by hanging at Brixton prison. He was mentally ill, with known suicidal tendencies, and his personal representatives sued for negligence. A number of allegations were made which included the defendants' failure to provide a proper system, proper staff and facilities for the care of the deceased, and failing to take proper care of his safety. The main thrust of the plaintiffs' case was that the defendants were negligent because the general standard of care provided in the prison was inadequate. The standard of care in the prison hospital should have been the same as that in a psychiatric hospital outside prison, and it fell below that standard. This argument was rejected by the judge and no negligence was found in this case. Mr Justice Pill stated:

> In making the decision as to the standard to be demanded the court must, however, bear in mind as one factor that resources available for the public service are limited and that the allocation of resources is a matter for Parliament. . . . Even in a medical situation outside prison, the standard of care required will vary with the context. The facilities available to deal with an emergency in a general practitioner's surgery cannot be expected to be as ample as those available in the casualty department of a general hospital, for example. . . . The duty is tailored to the act and function to be performed.

It is possible to agree with Mr Justice Pill's approximation of the standard of care in the case. Prison hospitals and specialist psychiatric hospitals perform different functions with different facilities and missions. However, the judge's reference to public services and Parliament's function does cause some concern. The judge did appear to be quite influenced by these factors. His comments are in marked contrast to the sentiments expressed by Lord Justice Mustill in the Bull case and in another case, *Wilsher v. Essex Area Health Authority*, [1986] 3 All ER 801.

The slippery slope for judges to avoid is that of sanctioning reductions in standards of care in public sector hospitals because Parliament controls their resources and these are limited. All hospitals open for public service should provide, in Lord Justice Dillon's words from the Bull case, 'a staff reasonably sufficient for the foreseeable requirements of the patient'. Lack of resources should not prevent the reasonable and safe provision of treatment. A hospital unit or ward which cannot provide 'a staff reasonably sufficient for the foreseeable requirements of the patient' should, arguably, close until it is able to do so, otherwise a potentially negligent healthcare system is primafacie in operation.

Brooks v. Home Office [1999] 2 FLR 33 helps clarify this issue of the standard of care in prison environments and environments of care generally. *Knight
v. Home Office* [1990] 3 All ER 237 was considered in the case. This case
involved a high-risk pregnancy remand prisoner in Holloway prison who was
expecting twins. A series of ultrasound scans were carried out by a variety
of different people. A scan performed when the prisoner was 36 weeks pregnant showed that one of the twins had not grown as expected since the previous scan, two weeks before. The prison contacted the local antenatal
clinic, but made an appointment for five day's time rather than requiring an
emergency appointment. Two days later, only one foetal heartbeat could be
detected and the prisoner was transferred to hospital. One twin was delivered stillborn; the other lived but later suffered complications, which
resulted in serious disability. The prisoner alleged that the prison had been
negligent in not transferring her immediately after the scan and in failing to
recognise and respond to the features of inter-uterine growth retardation.

The Home Office, responsible for the prison, argued that in deciding the
relevant standard of care, the court was entitled to take into account the fact
that the prisoner was in custody. Mr Justice Pill's judgment in *Knight v. Home
Office* [1990] 3 All ER 237 was considered by Mr Justice Garland and he
stated:

> I cannot regard Knight as authority for the proposition that the plaintiff
> should not, while detained in Holloway, be entitled to expect the same
> level of antenatal care, both for herself and her unborn infants, as if
> she were at liberty, subject of course to the constraints of having to
> be escorted and, to some extent, movements being retarded by those
> requirements.

Insufficient expertise could not defend failure to provide appropriate care.
The judge further stated: 'if a properly informed decision cannot be made
due to lack of experience or lack of information, the matter should be referred
to somebody capable of making that informed decision'.

The non-specialist medical staff at the prison should have referred the prisoner to a specialist unit immediately. The plaintiff lost her case on the issue
of causation. Expert evidence at the trial suggested that a two-day delay in
obtaining specialist advice would not have been a breach of duty. Therefore,
the stillbirth was not caused by any breach of duty, and no damages would
be awarded. This case is helpful in that it clarifies the Knight case. Knight
did not advance different and lower standards of medical care for prisoners. On its own particular facts, the Knight case makes sense. However,
the judge in the Brooks case was not prepared to advance it beyond those
facts. As Jones (2002) argues: 'Knight was distinguished on the basis that
it was concerned with the level of supervision for convicted prisoners with
psychiatric problems and a propensity to self-harm.'

Managers and staff are between a rock and a hard place in the poor resource
situation and there are no easy answers to the problems raised. This discussion

has focused on the area where it has been alleged that there was negligence in resource organisation and allocation, which resulted in patient injury. The term 'healthcare resource' has a wide meaning and includes medical and nursing staff as well as plant and equipment failing.

Conclusion

This chapter has discussed the concept of accountability within the current healthcare environment and negligence law. It is an environment which attempts to put the patient at the centre of the NHS. The concept of accountability can now be seen to exist alongside other concepts such as patient empowerment and clinical governance. Today, accountability is not such a new topic and to an extent, is seen as an implicit part of the care equation. Accountability 'has come home'.

It is possible to see some mixed messages coming from the courts when all the healthcare organisation negligent resource cases are considered together. The courts appear to be treading very carefully, but will not be afraid to challenge a decision in appropriate circumstances. Healthcare resources must be organised reasonably to be within the law. The concept of reasonableness does, however, allow them a fair degree of latitude in their decision making. The courts do maintain an important potential to safeguard patients' rights and interests in the NHS. They resolve disputes when called upon to do so, and through that process set legal principles, which provide a broad framework for decision making.

Chapter 6
Accountability and Clinical Governance: a Policy Perspective

Tracey Heath

Introduction

Each of the last three decades has brought with it an increasingly loud call to account. A call, which although arguably reflecting broader societal change, appears to have had a definite and concrete impact upon healthcare and the way in which it is developed, delivered, monitored and evaluated. In particular, organisational accountability for clinical care is no longer implicit, it is an explicit requirement underlined by the 'bold type' of policy documents. This chapter explores the impact of UK Government policy upon accountability, tracing its early manifestation in the audit society and individualism of the 1980s and early 1990s to the clinical governance agenda of today.

Background: the NHS pre-1997

1948 saw the advent of the UK National Health Service (NHS) – a service free to all at the point of delivery. Not unreasonably, although possibly naively given the benefit of hindsight, the thought had been that demand for and therefore the cost of healthcare would decrease as disease was controlled and the general health and circumstances of the population improved. However, expenditure continued to spiral upwards as public demand increased and the nature and variety of treatments available expanded.

Successive UK Governments have therefore been faced with the constant struggle to negotiate an acceptable balance between capitalising upon advances in research and technology (what could be done) on the one side and finite resources (what could be afforded) on the other. Unsurprisingly therefore, given the context of an ageing population and at times an ailing economy, the efficiency of the NHS has been high on the political agenda for several decades.

Concern for efficiency is nothing new: in many ways this had been a constant theme since the inception of the NHS. However it was not until the 1980s that it became a dominant policy issue. The then Conservative Government commissioned a rapid, independent review of the situation and the Griffiths Report was the result (Griffiths, 1983).

Griffiths had suggested that if Florence Nightingale were to carry her lamp through the corridors of the NHS she would be searching for those in charge. Given this background, the resulting recommendations were of little surprise. The principles of general management were viewed as the remedy to the organisation's problems, in particular the perceived lack of clarity regarding accountability at the local level. A new management structure was introduced from the top to the bottom of the NHS and almost immediately general managers, many of whom were from outside the public sector, were appointed on a performance-related basis. The challenge to professional autonomy was explicit: nurses lost the right to be managed by a member of their own profession, and their credibility as potential general managers was questioned. In turn, the right of medical practitioners to be shielded from questions regarding their use of the NHS' finite resources was also questioned (Spurgeon, 1997; Klein, 2001).

There had been high hopes that a system of general management would stem the tide of rising expenditure. Unfortunately, at least from a financial point of view, the Griffiths Report did not lead to the startling revolution in the functioning of the health service that was at first envisioned. However the next initiative, introduced in 1989 by the White Paper *Working for Patients* (Department of Health, 1989), was to have a much more profound impact.

Working for Patients separated purchaser and provider roles in healthcare and gave general practitioners the option of becoming fundholders. The internal market and associated changes thereby created were presented as part of a continued drive to decentralise the NHS and place responsibility for decision making, as much as possible, at the local level. This is of course arguable: the NHS was becoming more national than at the time of its inception, with one unified management structure in contrast to the disparate collection of different services it once was. The simulated market which was introduced brought with it pseudo consumerism and a collection of monitoring processes intended to reflect the performance of the various components of healthcare, and thereby inform decisions regarding the purchase and provision of services.

The reasoning behind these changes appeared sound: the money should follow the patient, therefore promoting rather than penalising productivity, as had previously been the case. It is no coincidence that during the late 1980s hospital doctors and general practitioners were required to participate in clinical audit and the Royal College of Nursing became a strong advocate of similar clinically driven quality improvement activities. As Manigan (1993) so aptly put it, nurses (and by implication other healthcare professionals) needed to demonstrate their worth if they wanted to remain as valued clinicians, teachers and managers. The term the 'audit society' is sometimes used to refer to this period and the flurry of measurement activity that accompanied it (Power, 2000).

Gray (2001) argues that throughout the 1980s and early 1990s the emphasis was on doing things correctly, both better (quality assurance) and more cheaply (efficiency), and that it has only been more recently that doing the right things (effectiveness) has been a major concern. Certainly Walsh (2000) argues that accountability for the quality of clinical care, and here we can assume its effectiveness, was something that was predominantly seen as the concern of individual clinicians rather than the organisation as a whole. This is a philosophy perhaps best embodied in nursing and midwifery by the 1992 *Code of Professional Conduct* (UKCC, 1992a) with its promotion of individual accountability for practice. It is worthy of note that in its recent revised form, attention is paid to the context within which individuals work (NMC, 2002b).

In 1996 the Conservatives attempted to bring new life into audit and other quality improvement activities with the publication of *Promoting Action on Clinical Effectiveness* (NHSE, 1996). Health authorities were made responsible for auditing the performance of NHS trusts and attempts were made to promote evidence-based practice through substantial investment in research and development, the production of guidance and outcome indicators. Much of the success of these initiatives relied upon the co-operation and professional ethos of the medical profession rather than demands from the centre for their compliance. Unfortunately, and some would say prematurely, they were replaced by the incoming Labour Government's more directive based approach before they were put to the test.

The Labour Government's challenge

On assuming office in 1997 the Labour Government inherited a complex set of challenges. On the one hand the 1990s had brought with it a loss of public confidence in the health service, poorly performing healthcare practitioners and seemingly unjustifiable variations in practice between regions. On the other hand this was accompanied by a history of previous substantial investment in research and development, audit, clinical effectiveness, risk management, and continuing professional development, and, no matter how generous Government spending, a finite budget to support any change (Table 6.1). For decades there appears to have been a constant swing between policies that promote central as opposed to devolved decision making in the NHS. This reflects the tensions inherent in the organisation. On the one hand its dependence on public funds centralises accountability, on the other the perceived inadequacy of those funds inevitably persuades ministers that it would be best to devolve responsibility for how they are spent (Klein, 2001).

Given this context, how was the Labour Government to respond? A complex task lay ahead, but what Labour did promise was that in its efforts to address these shortfalls there would be no return to the old centralised

Table 6.1   Driving policy: the Labour Government's challenge.

Key policy drivers	Illustrated by:
Loss of public confidence in the NHS	1996 50% of those interviewed declared themselves to be dissatisfied with the NHS (Mulligan, 1998)
Poorly performing healthcare practitioners	A rising number of complaints going to litigation (Department of Health, 1996) The number of cases that received high profile media coverage. For example: the Allitt enquiry a bone tumour service in Birmingham that misdiagnosed cancer, which in some cases led to unnecessary, drastic and disfiguring surgery errors in population screening programmes for women's cancers at Kent & Canterbury Hospital high death rates from paediatric heart surgery at Bristol (Donaldson & Gray, 1998; Brocklehurst & Walshe, 1999)
Variations in practice	Claims of 'postcode prescribing' In 1997 the Department of Heath reported variations in treatment patterns between regions (and even within regions). For example: the number of hip replacements in people aged over 65 varies from 10 to 51 per 10 000 of the population the proportion of women aged 25–64 screened for cervical cancer varies from 67% to 93% in different areas of the country (Department of Health, 1997)
Previous substantial investment in quality improvement initiatives	*First Department of Health Research and Development Strategy* (Department of Health, 1991) *The Culyer Report* (Department of Health, 1994a) made proposals to strengthen the quality of research and development and to protect its funding. *Evolution of NHS framework for risk management* (NHSE 1996a) NHSE(1996b) *Promoting Clinical Effectiveness: a framework for action in and through the NHS.* Policy initiatives such as *The Health of the Nation* (Department of Health, 1992).
Finite budget	Claims of under funding and the continued drive for efficiency. In 1996 the NHS was declared the people's top priority for extra spending (Mulligan, 1998)

command and control system. Furthermore, there was a pledge to save and modernise the NHS with a central commitment to 'what works' rather than any particular political ideology (Klein, 2001).

Practising within an era of increasing accountability

Before examining Labour's response to the challenges of improving clinical care it is helpful to look at the related key development of corporate governance.

Corporate governance

Originally established to protect shareholders' investments and company assets from fraud and malpractice, the principles of corporate governance were introduced into the NHS in 1994 as part of the Conservative Government's attempt to demonstrate their commitment to improving public services (Department of Health, 1994a). Interestingly, during the same period a number of financial irregularities had already started to come to light in the NHS (Smith, 1998). In the NHS, corporate governance is about having efficient and effective systems in place to show that those services provided are value for money and moreover, that public money is not wasted. The key principles underpinning corporate governance are:

- Accountability – everything done by those who work in the NHS must be able to stand the test of parliamentary scrutiny, public judgements on propriety and professional codes of conduct.

- Probity – an absolute standard of honesty in dealing with NHS assets: integrity should be the hallmark of all personal conduct in decisions affecting patients, staff and suppliers, and in the use of information acquired in the course of NHS duties.

- Openness – there should be sufficient transparency about NHS activities to promote confidence between the NHS authority or trust and its staff, patients and the public.   (Department of Health, 1994a, p. 2)

In short, corporate governance is about ensuring that public assets are not put at risk or public money wasted in the delivery of healthcare and in so doing it demands accountability, honesty and transparency in all activities. These principles would later be adopted by the Labour Government and re-emerge in policy documents intended to tackle the perceived decline in the reputation of the NHS and for standards of clinical care.

Towards a modern and dependable NHS: the Labour Government's response

Reflecting upon the challenges the NHS presented to the Labour Government when they came into power in 1997, review and modernisation of the healthcare system was almost inevitable. The drivers for change were strong and there was a political imperative to act. The 'new' way forward to a 'modern' NHS was revealed in the 1997 policy document: *The New NHS: Modern, Dependable* (Department of Health, 1997). Six key principles were identified:

- renewing the NHS as a genuinely national service
- making the delivery of healthcare against national standards a local responsibility
- getting the NHS to work in partnership
- driving efficiency
- focusing on quality
- rebuilding public confidence

The message was clear, the efficiency and effectiveness of the UK NHS and the clinical care it delivered needed to be increased, even if this meant (despite earlier reassurances to the contrary) reversing the previous drift towards decentralisation to an NHS much more strongly influenced by central Government.

Enter clinical governance

First introduced in 1998 clinical governance was described as:

> a framework through which NHS organisations are accountable for continuously improving the quality of their services and safeguarding high standards of care by creating an environment in which excellence in clinical care will flourish. (Department of Health, 1998, p. 33)

Clinical governance built upon its predecessor corporate governance and became an integral part of the NHS following the NHS Act of 1999.

As a result the last few years appear to have been dedicated to fathoming out what clinical governance is and how it can be made to work. Arguably, rather less attention has been given to whether it is a worthwhile endeavour. Clinical governance is associated with improving quality and as such, it is difficult to argue with; indeed to do so would appear morally unjust. Generally speaking most clinical staff have accepted the concept, if only as a result of the belief that problems with the NHS, that are currently largely (and one assumes incorrectly) attributed to failing healthcare professionals, will be exposed. That said, as a method to assure and improve quality, based upon accountability, it is not without its critics (Goodman, 1998; Loughlin, 2000). What does seem certain, however, is that the quality of clinical care has taken, and is set to remain, centre stage at least for the foreseeable future.

So what does clinical governance mean for individuals, practitioners and local organisations such as NHS trusts? From a very pragmatic standpoint many of the elements of clinical governance are 'nothing new'. Clinical governance is intended to promote the delivery of safe, effective, patient centred healthcare and encompasses many pre-existing systems and processes for monitoring and improving practice and services. Examples of such systems and processes include: clinical audit, risk management, education, training, continuing personal and professional development, and staffing and staff management.

However, greater emphasis is now placed upon involvement of patients and service users and the integration of existing quality initiatives to form a coherent whole. Gone are the days when departments such as risk management, audit and training could operate in relative isolation (if in fact they ever did so successfully). Integration and working together are seen as the keys to high quality healthcare. It is also recognised that co-operation rather than the competition of previous years (and reinforced through the internal market) must be promoted, if individuals and organisations are to share best practice and learn from each other's mistakes. This leads to the crux of the change: what clinical governance appears to represent, moreover require, is a whole cultural shift from a situation where when things went wrong the question asked was '*who* was to blame?' to one where the major challenge is to find out '*what* went wrong?'

The requirement for a 'no blame' culture and more integrated working arrangements are not the only major changes associated with clinical governance (Figure 6.1). For the first time since the inception of the NHS in 1948, accountability for the quality of clinical care rests firmly at organisational level; final legal responsibility being placed with the chief executives of NHS trusts (Department of Health, 1998).

Accountability and clinical governance

Organisational accountability

The emphasis of accountability at the corporate or organisational level has in the past focused largely upon financial duties and meeting certain workload or performance targets. Quality of care was a declared part of the corporate role, but in reality responsibility has rested almost exclusively at clinical rather than managerial level (Donaldson & Gray, 1998). The contracting process best illustrates this. Although contracts between purchasers and providers, introduced as part of the internal market in the 1990s, were intended to offer a way of making explicit expectations about the quality of services to be delivered, it is debatable whether the process operated as intended. For example, Gray and Donaldson (1996) found little evidence to suggest that there was a systematic approach to promoting and assuring quality when contracts were drawn up.

On assuming power in 1997, the Labour Government lost little time in making clinical quality (through clinical governance) a statutory requirement at the local level. The four main components of clinical governance for health service trusts were spelled out in *A first class service* (Department of Health, 1998). NHS trusts were expected to demonstrate:

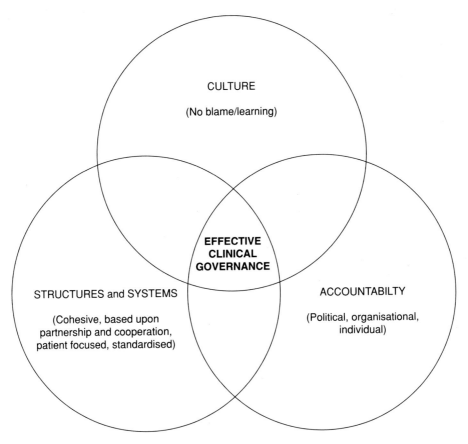

Figure 6.1   Effective clinical governance: dominant policy themes.

- clear lines of accountability and responsibility for the quality of services
- an extensive programme of quality improvement initiatives and activities
- clear policies aimed at managing risks
- procedures for all professional groups to identify and remedy poor performance in all professional groups.

The organisation's chief executive was given ultimate responsibility for assuring the quality of services provided and a designated senior clinician (usually the medical or nursing director) was charged with ensuring that systems were in place to support clinical governance and to monitor effectiveness. Formal arrangements for trust boards to discharge their responsibilities for clinical quality were required and an annual reporting process instituted.

A concept allied to clinical governance is that of controls assurance. Based upon best governance practice (NHSE, 1999b), controls assurance completes the governance picture by assuring, through the introduction of

18 standards, the quality of non-clinical support services such as health and safety and waste management. By doing so it recognises that the success of processes to maximise clinical and non-clinical quality are to some extent interdependent.

Clinical governance, which is essentially about accountable and dependable local delivery of clear national standards of service, is unsurprisingly also monitored by the centre. The Commission for Health Improvement (CHI) was established to perform just such a function, and builds upon the work of other monitoring strategies such as the national performance framework and national patient and user survey (Department of Health, 1997/1998).

CHI was established to support and scrutinise local clinical governance arrangements independently through scheduled programmes of review. Originally depicted as a watchdog not dissimilar to the Office for Standards in Education (OFSTED), more recent conceptualisations have portrayed a more developmental, softer touch organisation. Nonetheless there are some similarities between CHI and OFSTED. It has statutory powers and is accountable to Government for its work, although operating independently and collaborating with other bodies such as the Royal Colleges, regulatory and voluntary organisations (OFSTED, 2002; Department of Health, 1997/1998, CHI, 2001).

CHI is keen to emphasise that the patient experience is at the heart of its work. Its main functions are said to be:

- to independently scrutinise the local clinical governance arrangements of NHS trusts
- to conduct or assist in the investigation of serious service failures and intervention to put things right
- to monitor and review the implementation of national service frameworks, National Institute for Clinical Excellence (NICE) guidance and other key NHS policy priorities
- to provide leadership, identify and share best practice related to clinical governance   (adapted from CHI, 2001)

Accountability implies visibility. Walsh (2000) argues that nurses cannot be accountable unless there are unambiguous outcomes and standards against which performance can be measured. His point, that expectations must be clear if one is to be expected to explain how or why they have not been met, would appear to apply equally well at an organisational level too. NHS trusts could reasonably expect to be informed of the remit for which they are required to account. The 'bold type' of Government policy makes this clear too. Arguably the guidance produced by NICE, the publication of national service frameworks and performance indicators, and clear policy priorities serve to fulfil this function. Organisations know they will be measured, know what they will be measured against and furthermore what they will be expected to account for if they are perceived to fall short of requirements.

Individual accountability

The implication of the above changes in organisational accountability for individual practitioners is not difficult to calculate. The success of the clinical governance process demands that the responsibilities and sphere of accountability of individuals within an organisation are explicit too. Put simply, as a chief executive with ultimate responsibility for clinical quality, most of us would wish to ensure that doctors, nurses and other healthcare professionals were clear on the role they were required to fulfil in order to make the organisation a success. That said, accountability is a two-way process. Those holding nurses to account must remember their half of the contract and make sure the resources (whether equipment or training and education) and authority are available to allow them to function in an accountable manner. This responsibility, which has received limited attention in the past, appears to have been underlined by recent reforms.

In reality then, accountability can occur at different levels. For example, in the event of a serious incident resulting from failure to follow identified best practice, organisations would be expected to account for the structure and systems they have in place to support the dissemination and execution of best practice. However, individual clinicians would be expected to account for their decision to employ or reject the use of a particular practice or intervention in an individual case.

Political accountability

There is no doubt that NHS trust chief executives face two very daunting tasks. First, in ensuring that requirements associated with financial accountability and clinical accountability do not come in to conflict. Second, in fostering a no blame culture in a climate where the personal and professional accountability of individual employees is explicitly reinforced.

At first sight it would appear that responsibility and accountability for the quality of clinical care rests solely at the local level and that the Government have somehow managed to distance themselves from public accountability in all but their role as the monitor, evaluator and reporter of progress. However, an alternative view is possible. As discussed earlier, successive Governments have striven to achieve a balance between devolution and central control. Whilst the 'how' of clinical governance is to some extent left to local interpretation (although even this is subject to question given the level of detail provided by central guidance) the Government appears to have retained a great deal of authority and power over NHS trusts. In fact Government policy, through national service frameworks and the work of NICE and CHI, has extended its influence into areas previously regarded as the exclusive domain of managers and clinicians.

Accountability involves responsibility, knowledge and being able to justify your actions. It also involves the ability to make decisions and carry them through into practice – autonomy and authority (Walsh, 2000). In exercising a greater degree of central control over practice and services, the

Government must accept some accountability for clinical quality. Thus whilst the quality reforms in general terms have served to emphasise both the accountability of individual professionals and the organisations for which they work, they can equally be viewed as making policy makers more explicitly accountable too. By taking greater control, policy makers have also assumed greater responsibility for clinical performance, and made it more difficult for any distinction to be drawn between the domains of policy and practice in the future (Walshe *et al.*, 2000). This is good news when things are progressing well, less so when healthcare is perceived to be in decline.

Reflections on the broader policy context

On initial inspection the Labour Government's response to the problems of the NHS, i.e. the emergence of clinical governance and associated policy developments, appears to be logical, in fact almost predictable (Table 6.2).

Table 6.2   The new policy agenda.

Key policy drivers	The new policy agenda	Illustrative publications
Loss of public confidence in the NHS	Greater public involvement in service and practice development and the process of professional self-regulation. Open and honest communication regarding performance, and how mistakes have been managed and learned from	Department of Health (1997) *The new NHS: modern, dependable*, Department of Health (1998) *Quality in the new NHS*, Department of Health (2000c) *An organisation with a memory*
Poorly performing healthcare practitioners	Strengthened and more equitable professional self-regulation Recognition that professional bodies such as the Nursing & Midwifery Council only form part of the regulatory framework and need to be supplemented by other national (NICE, NSF, CHI) and local bodies (procedures to tackle poor performance, speaking out policies, no blame culture) Modernising pre-registration education and training Targeted and coordinated continuing professional development Recruiting and retaining experienced clinical staff	Department of Health (2000b) *The NHS plan*, Department of Health (1999e) *Making a difference*, NHSE (2000) *Modernising regulation: the new nursing and midwifery council*

Table 6.2 *(cont'd)*

Key policy drivers	The new policy agenda	Illustrative publications
Variations in practice	Promoting and supporting a more standardised approach to treatment and care through investment in robust research and development, mechanisms to support evidence-based practice and the application of consistent quality standards across the service (through the introduction of NICE, CHI, National Benchmarks etc.) Emphasis on sharing, partnership and cooperation rather than competition and the subsequent demise of the internal market	Department of Health (1997) *The new NHS: modern, dependable*, Department of Health (1998) *Quality in the new NHS,* Department of Health (2001f) *Research Governance Framework for Health & Social Care*
Previous substantial investment in quality improvement initiatives	Quality as everyone's business Coordination and targeting of activities through national priorities Clinical governance and its emphasis upon accountability and 'joined-up thinking' Working across professional boundaries and blurring roles Monitoring to ensure things work (for example, through CHI, National Patient and User Survey, National performance indicators, existing accreditation schemes, controls assurance) Freedom of organisations to run own affairs linked to progress in establishing clinical governance Modernisation	Department of Health (1997) *The new NHS: modern, dependable*, Department of Health (1998a) *Quality in the new NHS*, Department of Health (2000b) *The NHS plan*
Finite budget	Emphasis on efficient use of resources Emphasis upon proper regulation of financial affairs (corporate governance) Recognition that change will not happen instantly and the need for a ten-year plan of investment and reform	Department of Health (1997) *The new NHS: modern, dependable*, Department of Health (1994a) *Corporate governance in the NHS*, Department of Health (2000) *The NHS Plan*

Many of the initiatives build upon the work of the previous Conservative Government, whilst providing added emphasis on the need for cohesiveness (joined-up thinking), partnership as opposed to competition, accountability, openness and public involvement (Figure 6.1). And although there is some variation in detail between countries, similar expectations of quality and efficiency and accountability have developed across the UK. For example, the NHS in Scotland has established the Clinical Standards Board for Scotland with a remit not dissimilar to CHI (Clinical Standards Board for Scotland, 2002).

However, just as the introduction of clinical governance cannot be viewed in isolation from the introduction of NICE, NSFs and CHI, so, too, broader policy initiatives cannot be ignored. The NHS does not operate in isolation. Strengthened systems of professional self-regulation and professional education, in addition to corporate governance have all served to play a part in reinforcing the process of accountable healthcare (Table 6.2). It is doubtful whether any of the measures would provide the key to safe, effective and affordable healthcare if employed singularly, but together the Government's reforms provide a comprehensive policy framework, a strong feature of which appears to be 'control'. Mandating quality improvement through central policy has not been particularly successful in the past, either in the UK or abroad (Walshe *et al.*, 2000). Effective governance requires a cultural change and, as the Government appears to have realised, a realignment of incentives and other policy issues (of particular note in this respect is the abolition of the internal market).

Conclusion

In this brief analysis of the policy context surrounding the introduction of clinical governance and associated quality reforms, there are four main conclusions:

- New Labour is in many ways building upon the policies of the earlier Conservative Governments. Despite the emphasis upon the new, much of the old that worked has been retained.
- Clinical governance requires a cultural shift and poses significant challenges for both local organisations and individual clinicians.
- Accountability is considered central to the success of clinical governance and in turn the delivery of safe and effective healthcare.
- There is tension between the desire to strengthen the grip of central Government and the need for devolution and democracy.

An interesting compromise has resulted; only time will tell whether the correct balance between individual and organisational accountability and political control has been struck.

Chapter 7

Accountability in NHS Trusts
Stephen Knight and Tony Hostick

Introduction

All healthcare professionals, including nurses, are accountable for their clinical practice and this is demonstrated by compliance with clinical standards, professional codes and standards, and the law. The UKCC and its successor organisation the NMC, have, through successive issues of a *Code of Professional Conduct* (UKCC, 1992a; NMC, 2002b) made accountability for practice explicit for registered nurses. In addition, practitioners are accountable for meeting the contractual obligations set by employers who expect quality healthcare to be delivered by employees within a clinical policy framework. The interest of the law is that nurses and midwives act in the best interest and for the protection of individuals and the general public.

However, accountability is not only within the domain of the individual. The nursing profession, through the NMC, and formerly the UKCC, is itself accountable, as are employing organisations, who as employers are accountable in law and more recently through clinical governance arrangements within NHS organisations.

This chapter summarises the principles of accountability within the context of clinical governance and professional self-regulation. A stepped approach to decision making will be outlined and some of the implications for nursing practice and organisations are explored.

Clinical governance

In recent years, extensive media coverage of significant failures in clinical practice has resulted in a rise in public and political concern regarding maintenance of safety in healthcare delivery. This concern has resulted in the UK Government deciding that it is no longer willing to accept that professions can, in isolation, be relied upon to regulate their own practice and decision making. Whilst stopping short of withdrawing the right of healthcare professions to regulate themselves, changes have been made to ensure that monitoring of practice and, where necessary, corrective action is taken to ensure patient safety.

Probably the most significant, far reaching and potentially culture changing decision by the Government was to make NHS chief executives responsible for ensuring the quality of professional decision making and the management of care in their organisation. Through this decision, NHS trusts became accountable for ensuring quality in healthcare delivery (Department of Health, 1997) and clinical governance was born. The implementation of local clinical governance arrangements has been determined to be the vehicle through which quality will be delivered (Department of Health, 1998a). The key concept here is quality, which Lilley (1999, p. ix) defines as:

> knowing what outcome you want and being sure you get it, every time, for as long as you want it . . . quality is not just a process. It is an outcome and has its foundation in consistency. Plus, it can be changed, upgraded or dumped for something better.

Quality is not measured on a static scale but can change according to context, individual and public perception and the acquisition of new knowledge.

The World Health Organisation (1983) divides quality into four components:

- professional performance (technical quality)
- resource use (efficiency)
- risk management (the risk of injury or illness associated with the service provided)
- patients' satisfaction with the service provided

The principles of clinical governance are not new and reflect the World Health Organisation's components of quality outlined above. Clearly those four aspects of quality underpin the concept of clinical governance, which has been defined as:

> a framework through which NHS organisations are accountable for continuously improving the quality of their services and safeguarding high standards of care by creating an environment in which excellence in clinical care will flourish. (Department of Health, 1998)

The Government's vision of a framework for quality included:

- clear national evidence set by the National Service Frameworks (NSFs) and National Institute for Clinical Excellence (NICE)
- local delivery of quality services
- monitoring of services through the Commission for Health Improvement (CHI)
- consultation with patients and the public

Responsibilities of trusts

Through the clinical governance framework, healthcare professions and individual practitioners within NHS organisations are responsible and accountable for the provision of 'best practice', as is the chief executive of each NHS organisation. In fact, as Lilley points out:

> Clinical governance builds on the idea that quality is everyone's responsibility – we can all play our part. The patient's passage through an episode of sickness that takes them back to wellness involves scores of people. The car park attendant and the consultant surgeon, from the cleaner across to the community nurse, we all have a part to play. (Lilley, 1999, p. vi)

Accountability in the NHS relies upon evidence of fulfilment of responsibilities by individuals, professional bodies and NHS organisations themselves. The achievement of clinical governance is to a large degree also dependent on the application of other concepts including professional self-regulation, user involvement/participation, evidence-based practice and lifelong learning.

The Commission for Health Improvement (CHI) was established by the Government to assure and monitor improvement in the quality of patient care by undertaking clinical governance reviews. The framework for reviews adopted by CHI provides a useful outline of the technical components of clinical governance and the related responsibilities of NHS organisations (Commission for Health Improvement, 2002). Scrutiny of these components and related responsibilities will help clarify how NHS trusts are expected to demonstrate accountability.

The technical components of clinical governance, sometimes known as the 'seven pillars of clinical governance' are:

- risk management
- patient and public involvement
- clinical audit
- clinical effectiveness
- staffing and staff management
- education, training and continuing professional development
- use of information

Each of these components is assessed by CHI review teams in terms of five themes, or groups of responsibilities for which NHS organisations are accountable. The five themes are:

- accountabilities and structures
- strategies and plans
- application of policies, strategies and plans
- quality improvements and learning
- resources and training for staff

NHS trusts are accountable to the Department of Health, through newly formed strategic health authorities, for ensuring that each of the five themes are applied to the seven technical components to identify, plan, implement and monitor areas for improvement in quality of care.

Accountabilities and structures

NHS trusts are required to be able to demonstrate that measures are in place for ensuring that their responsibilities for each of the seven technical components are met. Each trust is expected to develop a committee structure for clinical governance that ensures development of strategies for quality improvement, identifies the responsibilities of staff and encourages monitoring of activities by management teams. It is therefore typical of most trusts that committees exist for such things as risk management, audit, education and training, health and safety. These committees usually report to a quality and clinical governance committee which is a sub-committee of, and therefore accountable to, the NHS trust board.

Strategies and plans

Trusts must be able to demonstrate at all times that comprehensive strategies and implementation plans are in place for the management of each of the seven components of clinical governance. One of these areas is risk management. A wide-ranging discussion of risk is not possible within the scope of this chapter. Therefore, a brief exploration of the concept of risk and its management may be useful in demonstrating the necessity for development and implementation of effective strategies and plans.

Risk has been defined in a variety of ways. However, according to Alaszewski (2000, p. 5) risk is composed of three underlying elements:

- consequences of actions
- the probability of different types of consequences
- the intentions of individuals involved.

Since health services are usually concerned with achieving specified outcomes, Alaszewski believes that the concept of intention should be included in a definition of risk in relation to healthcare delivery and defines risk in this context as: 'the possibility that a course of action will not achieve its desired and intended outcome but instead some unexpected situation will develop' (Alaszewski, 2000, p. 4). The new governing body, the NMC has identified in the revised *Code of Professional Conduct* that: 'As a registered nurse or midwife, you must act to identify and minimise the risk to patients and clients' (Nursing and Midwifery Council, 2002b, p. 9).

However, the management of risk is not left entirely as a responsibility of the practitioner, as clinical governance principles require that NHS trusts put in place mechanisms for identifying and addressing both clinical and non-clinical risk. Hence, the profession sets out the requirement for individuals to participate actively in risk management but trusts provide the policies and guidelines that constitute a problem-solving framework for practitioners.

A strategy for risk management could be expected to include plans for integration of all clinical and non-clinical risk management activities, such as collation of information related to risk, assessment and identification of risk, incident reporting, complaints management, health and safety, and attainment of controls assurance standards. Consideration should also have been given to the development and dissemination of processes for decision making with regard to risk and to the involvement of patients, users and other agencies in the risk management process. Evidence-based protocols for risk management should be formulated and resources diverted to reduce risk, which may result in the development of specialist support, e.g. infection control teams and tissue viability teams.

Application of policies, strategies and plans
A key feature of clinical governance is the monitoring of activities to ensure not only that policies and strategies are implemented but also that action plans to address particular issues are completed within agreed timescales to meet specific objectives. Such plans may result from local issues identified through audit, incident reporting or complaints management or may result from national concerns. A recent example of the latter is the Department of Health response to reports of death caused by errors in intrathecal (spinal) drug injections. In response to this issue, action plans for the management of intrathecal injection and the training of staff were issued to NHS trusts and monitored by the Department of Health to ensure that the problem is not repeated (Department of Health, 2001g).

An important factor in the monitoring of policies, strategies and plans by trusts is the maintenance of accurate systems that promote accurate record keeping and communication of information whilst maintaining confidentiality about patients/service users as required by the 1998 Data Protection Act. Whilst individual professionals are responsible for accurate record keeping, the development, implementation and maintenance of record systems is a corporate responsibility

Quality improvements and learning
A guiding principle of clinical governance is that lessons are learnt from change, management experience and involvement in quality initiatives. Trusts are now required to develop systems for dissemination and feedback to staff of lessons learnt from audit, staff and patient surveys, risk management activities and evidence-based practice.

Resources and training for staff
In order for staff to participate fully in clinical governance activities and thereby also exercise individual and professional accountability, NHS trusts should provide training and support for staff including:

- interpretation and support of clinical information
- management of information
- customer care
- risk prevention and management
- clinical audit

- literature, database and Internet search skills
- critical appraisal skills.

In summary, each NHS trust is responsible and accountable for providing a core infrastructure and resources to support individuals, comprising training and education, information or knowledge management, access to effective activity recording and management systems. Further to this, NHS trusts must demonstrate evidence-based managerial decision making by aggregating the information collected from individuals, teams and services to inform local needs and priorities. However, it might be said that the first responsibility of the organisation is to provide the time and resources for all of the above to take place.

Professional self-regulation

The purpose of professional self-regulation is the protection of the public through professional standards. Professional self-regulation is in fact a contract between the profession and the public, which allows professions to regulate their own members in order to protect the public from poor or unsafe practice (UKCC, 2001a). In exchange for the privilege of professional self-regulation nurses are obliged to practice within the NMC's code of professional conduct. In addition registered practitioners must monitor themselves and their colleagues in order to:

- promote good practice
- prevent poor practice
- intervene in unacceptable practice.

The *Code of Professional Conduct* (UKCC, 2001a) stated: 'the principles of professional self-regulation are inextricably linked to those underpinning clinical governance. Both professional self-regulation and clinical governance are the business of every registered practitioner'. It can be seen that the principles underpinning clinical governance and professional self-regulation are not only inextricably linked but indicate not only to whom nurses are accountable but how accountability might be demonstrated. The opening statement of the *Code of Professional Conduct* was explicit regarding accountability of the individual practitioner:

> Each registered nurse, midwife and health visitor shall act, at all times in such a manner as to safeguard and promote the interests of individual patients and clients, serve the interests of society, justify public trust and confidence and uphold the good standing and confidence of the profession.

The introduction of clinical governance responsibilities in NHS organisations has re-emphasised the need for accountability frameworks such as the one provided by the *Code of Professional Conduct*. Rather than replicate

Table 7.1 The principles for exercising accountability.

(1) The interests of the patient or client are paramount.
(2) Professional accountability must be exercised in such a manner as to ensure that the primacy of the interests of patients or clients is respected and must not be overridden by those of the professions or their practitioners.
(3) The exercise of accountability requires the practitioner to seek to achieve and maintain high standards.
(4) Advocacy on behalf of patients or clients is an essential feature of the exercise of accountability by a professional practitioner.
(5) The role of other persons in the delivery of healthcare to patients or clients must be recognised and respected, provided that the first principle above is honoured.
(6) Public trust and confidence in the profession is dependent on its practitioners being seen to exercise their accountability responsibly.
(7) Each registered nurse, midwife or health visitor must be able to justify any action or decision not to act taken in the course of their professional practice.

this code, for the purpose of this chapter it may be more useful to summarise the principles for exercising accountability in Table 7.1 (UKCC, 1989). Within the principles for exercising accountability outlined in Table 7.1 it is explicit that the first principle is paramount, and that any intervention should result in a benefit or advantage to the patient or client. Other key factors are achieving and maintaining high standards and recognising and respecting the roles of other persons in healthcare delivery.

The underpinning principle of clinical governance is a commitment to ensuring that people who receive services are involved at all levels of decision making within the NHS. Service users should have access to up-to-date, accurate information and should be encouraged to be reciprocal partners in their own care. Nurses and other professionals should be 'clinically effective' whenever possible and appropriate. Research findings that have been appraised using the 'hierarchy of evidence' (NHS Centre for Reviews and Dissemination, 1996) should be applied in practice. For individuals, clinical effectiveness means the degree to which a treatment achieves the health improvement for a patient that it is designed to achieve. For organisations, it means the degree to which the organisation is ensuring that 'best practice' is used wherever possible (CHI glossary of *Clinical Governance Reviews*, 2001).

It is considered that this definition is inadequate for the scope of nursing in particular and that elements other than treatment should also be considered including advice, care, therapy, palliation, non-clinical need, choice, risk, etc., which do not always lead to a demonstrable health improvement but do achieve other outcomes.

A systematic approach to decision making

The above principles illustrate the need for a systematic approach, as in the example outlined below. A standardised approach based on individual need with the potential for involving the patient or client, carers and others can be used to minimise problems and provide a framework for addressing dilemmas.

The nursing process (Christensen & Kenney, 1995) offers a broad, normative approach in terms of assessment, planning, implementation and evaluation. The first step in a systematic approach is assessment. For many disciplines this will be a predominantly clinical assessment. However, it can also include a needs assessment and a risk assessment. This will help formulate a diagnosis or problem. Based on the formulation, the next decision is to consider the most effective or appropriate intervention. Following the intervention, or establishing reasons for using alternative interventions, its effectiveness and patient satisfaction should be evaluated. Not only do nurses have to ensure that what they do is 'the right thing' they have to be seen to have done 'the right thing' by recording their actions effectively.

All of the above steps should be recorded accurately, legibly and completely as they occur (Department of Health, 1999b). If key decisions are recorded contemporaneously then a true and accurate record is available as evidence that will pass scrutiny under the requirements of the Bolam test (1957): in other words, the standard of care expected of the ordinary skilled person exercising and professing to have that special skill.

Implications for practice

Having outlined what should be done about the principles of professional accountability, how will this be achieved in practice? The challenges that face nurses today and the decisions that they take will all have consequences and inevitably pose problems or even dilemmas in practice. Likewise, the increased responsibilities of clinical governance will place extra demands on NHS trusts.

The following are some of the issues that need to be addressed. The intention is that readers can apply these questions to their own practice and develop responses that are meaningful to them and their situation. Through this they should be clearer about their personal development needs and be able to highlight areas for organisational action.

Assessment

How do you assess individual need, risk, and clinical state? Effective assessment should identify patient need. Sometimes this will be more apparent than on other occasions and range from relatively simple to extremely complex needs. For example, someone presenting with a simple trauma or wound through to a homeless, alcohol-dependent person with a learning disability, presenting with a head wound, florid hallucinations and threats of violence to others. Need will also depend on context of time, place and person: for example, presenting at night or during office hours, presenting at an A & E department or in the person's home, an individual's personality and traits, the experience and expertise of the nurse. Need could also be observed (signs), reported (symptoms) or masked (present yet unobserved or unreported).

Which tools do you use?
Which tool is right for the job? Is there a need for screening or triage? Do you use a generic global assessment measure or something more specific? Is it valid and reliable?

Involvement of users/carers/others
How do you engage and involve patients and carers? There needs to be appropriate levels of engagement and involvement based on simple or complex need. How much time do you have available? Assessment and interventions may be uni-disciplinary (simple) or require input from a number of different disciplines (complex). How easy is it to access complex care packages? Can all disciplines/agencies be engaged?

Evidence-based practice
Is any guidance available? If there is then how strong is the evidence base? According to the hierarchy of evidence then evidence from randomised controlled trials that are well designed and implemented should be utilised. However, to meet these requirements, then the problem, intervention and outcome indicators need to be clearly defined. Therefore, supporting evidence for discrete interventions to meet simple need is more likely to be available and to be more robust. It is in the areas of more complex need and multi-disciplinary interventions that convincing evidence is less likely to be available.

Are there any reasons not to follow guidance?
Any research, no matter how well designed and applied, will only suggest that something is relatively effective with some people some of the time. Therefore, although it may be the best option available, it needs to be considered against clinical experience and knowledge within what could be termed 'advanced practice'. If there is a reason to vary from the guidance then it will need to be recorded and justified. This is particularly important as clause 1.3 of the NMC *Code of Professional Conduct* states that: 'You (the practitioner) are accountable for your practice. This means that you are answerable for your actions and omissions, regardless of advice or directions from another professional' (Nursing and Midwifery Council, 2002b, p. 3). If there is no evidence, how urgently do you need to take the decision? Do you have time to find out? Do you have easy access to library information services? Can you find the evidence and appraise it? Is there someone who can do this for you?

Appropriate training and self-development
Should resources be invested to provide training and opportunities for everyone to be able to access, review and appraise evidence or should we invest in a service to produce evidence-based standards or a combination of both?

Many of the studies looking at the implementation of evidence into practice, for example, the Linear Model (Haines & Jones, 1994) and the Effective Health Care bulletin (NHS Centre for Reviews and Dissemination, 1999), seem to conclude that there are three critical requirements that need to be combined for success.

- high quality evidence, which needs to be operationally defined and incorporate research, consensus clinical experience, consumer experience (staff and patients)
- context, which requires a diagnostic of culture (barriers/enhancements), priorities, leadership, evaluation systems (clinical, economic, satisfaction), resources (time/people)
- skilled facilitation including the roles and skills associated with evaluator/researcher, educator/facilitator, change management, expert/opinion, leader

The contribution of reflective practice/supervision to accountability/minimising risk is also key. Time for reflection and the opportunity for effective clinical supervision using an appropriate framework is essential and should be an integral part of nurses' practice. How can you/the organisation find the time to do all this? Are the skills required readily available?

Ethics
Are there any ethical considerations to your decisions?

Conclusion

In summary this chapter has been concerned with accountability in NHS trusts and an attempt has been made to demonstrate the relationship between individual, professional and organisational accountability. Whilst professional requirements of the individual nurse continue to grow, NHS trusts also have a responsibility to ensure that the milieu in which professionals work is conducive to the provision of a quality service and that the quality of healthcare is monitored and continuously improved.

Chapter 8

Accountability and Clinical Governance in Nursing: a Manager's Perspective

Linda Pollock

Introduction

I have been a manager at director level for nearly 13 years, and so see, with the wonderful wisdom of retrospect, the many attempts made in the past decade or so to introduce 'quality controls', 'total quality management', 'quality assurance' and 'continuous quality improvement'. Often implemented on a 'top-down' basis, these quality initiatives received lip-service, and were often adopted with resigned cynicism by senior managers and practitioners alike (see Donaldson & Muir Gray's (1998) analysis of this topic). This has not been the case with the concept of clinical governance. It has been accepted wholeheartedly by an impressive number and range of 'leaders and followers' within the NHS.

Background context

I intend to focus on the Scottish system, so first of all will give a little bit of historical context. *Designed to Care*, the NHS White Paper produced at the end of 1997 by the new Labour Scottish Parliament, created our current structures (Scottish Executive Health Department, 1998). Each health board has two trusts, an acute trust and a primary care trust. (Exceptionally, Lothian, where I work, has a third trust, in West Lothian, where an integrated model of acute and primary care working is being piloted for the rest of Scotland.) The creation of two trusts per health board meant that there were fewer management units, and management costs were reduced. With *Designed to Care* there was abolition of the business-orientated, contract-orientated market environment in which we previously worked, and in its place we were encouraged to collaborate and bring down the barriers which impede effective communication and working together. GP fund-holding disappeared and in its place we have local healthcare co-operatives, or LHCCs.

With *Designed to Care* there was a re-affirmation of the Government's support of the NHS as a public service. More importantly perhaps, there was an emphasis on 'patient focus', developing effective services, and high quality care to patients (and carers) at every part of the patient's journey. This, in my view, is why the concept of clinical governance gained support from such a wide constituency, almost overnight.

Clinical governance as a concept

Designed to Care introduced the concept of clinical governance and shortly afterwards the Scottish Office issued national guidance to confirm that all trusts had to set up clinical governance systems (Scottish Executive Health Department, 1998). This guidance has been updated with the latest guidance being MEL (2000) 29 (Scottish Executive Health Department, 2000c). With the creation of unified health boards, set up in October 2001, a working paper on *New Governance Arrangements in NHS in Scotland* (Scottish Executive Health Department, 2001d) was produced. This guidance stated that a clinical governance standing committee should exist at unified health board level. Thus, clinical governance is here to stay and accountabilities pervade the new structures, to the very top. The term took over from the 'corporate governance' of the predecessor Government and has become central to how we work. I am sure that it is a term that will endure and we will hear a lot more about it in the years to come.

Some say that clinical governance is just new jargon, but the reality is that chief executives are now accountable for (though I must admit I thought they always were responsible for) the quality of service within their trusts. They now have to make sure that infrastructures exist within the trusts to ensure that clinical governance and quality systems are actually in place, and that quality of service provision is really happening. McSherry & Haddock (1999) illustrated clinical governance clearly (see Figure 8.1).

The meaning of clinical governance

'Clinical governance' is an umbrella term which requires us at trust board, i.e. at trust level, to produce evidence that we are: taking steps, first of all, to reduce the clinical risks that face the trust; taking steps to promote quality services and practice developments; encouraging clinical audit; and expanding research and development. We must make sure that the systems are in place so that all staff – especially, from my perspective as nursing director, that nurses – have access to research findings, that these research findings are disseminated, and that recommendations based on the research are implemented and monitored as appropriate. We want to continue to get evidence-based practice in place and we need to demonstrate this at trust board level. Ultimately we wish to ensure trust policies and guidelines are informed by the know-how and expertise of staff. We need to make sure too, that clinical policies are in place in line with local, national and

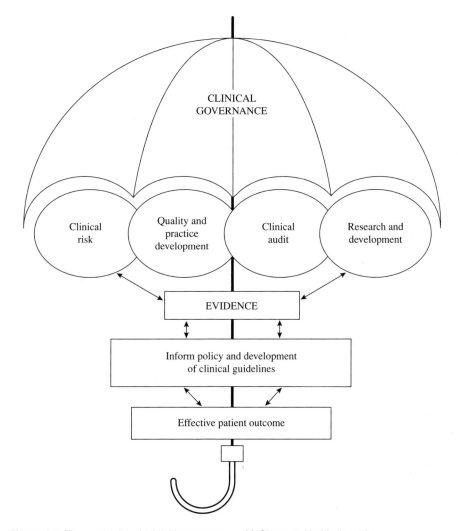

Figure 8.1 The umbrella of clinical governance. McSherry & Haddock, 1999.

international standards. The intention is that, as a result, patients will benefit and there will be improved outcomes for all who use the health service.

Our interpretation of clinical governance

Within the trust in which I work, a primary care trust, we have added two 'balloons' to Figure 8.1 – staff/people governance and public involvement. The first we added because, for us, quality service delivery is more than developing evidence-based protocols. It is also about valuing, supporting and training our staff. We believe that the best kept standards are those that are

Lothian Primary Care NHS Trust
CLINICAL GOVERNANCE COMMITTEE: MATRIX of CLINICAL GOVERNANCE STRANDS

CLINICAL EFFECTIVENESS	PUBLIC INVOLVEMENT	RISK MANAGEMENT

• Clinical Audit
• Clinical Guidelines
• Evidence-Based Practice
• Referral Protocols
• Information – Library/IT
	• Patient Information
	• Planning Services
	• Review of Services
	• Link Inequalities, Advocacy, Carers and Volunteering
		• CNORIS
		• Clinical Risk
		  – Resuscitation
		  – Infection Control
		  – Critical Incident Review
		• Confidentiality

RESEARCH and DEVELOPMENT • Increasing research capacity • Managing existing research grants • Encouraging new research • Maintaining ethical principles • Implementing research findings	**ACCREDITATION of SERVICE** • Clinical Standards Board for Scotland • Mental Welfare Commission • Scottish Health Advisory Service • Practice Accreditation • Investors in People • BS EN ISO 9001/2 • European Foundation Quality Model	**COMPLAINTS/LITIGATION** • Local resolution • Staff awareness • Informing patients and users • Learning from complaints
LIFELONG LEARNING • Training for Change • Continuing Personal Development	**PEOPLE GOVERNANCE** ACCREDITATION of PEOPLE • Appraisal • Revalidation	**MANAGING UNDER-PERFORMANCE/ SUPPORTING BEST PRACTICE**

(NOTE: Bullet points in each Strand Group are not intended to be exclusive nor comprehensive)

Figure 8.2 Matrix of clinical government strands, reproduced with permission from the Lothian Primary Care NHS Trust Clinical Governance Committee.

set by the staff and if the latter are supported to carry out quality work they will do so. Having this strand as an element of clinical governance highlighted the importance of work in this area and means that the trust board monitors progress and receives reports of action taken in relation to training, development and improving staff performance.

'Public involvement' is another 'balloon' that we have added below the umbrella. This represents the importance we ascribe to user and carer feedback in relation to service planning, development and redesign. We have a steering group that meets regularly to facilitate and encourage the development of a range of activities encompassed by 'user involvement'. We have also developed a trust public involvement strategy to give direction to this endeavour.

The approach which we have taken in my trust is summarised in the matrix shown in Figure 8.2.

Has clinical governance made a difference?

Clinical governance and its impact at board level

I believe that the introduction of clinical governance has made a difference, at a variety of levels. At trust board level, we were required to give clinical governance matters equal weight with business and financial matters. As a result, the trust board agenda is much more clinically focused. Board papers are regularly prepared on the strands of clinical governance – clinical risk, audit, research and development – and there is no doubt that the trust board is now focusing much more on service development and quality service provision. As a nursing director I regularly report and produce papers on nursing and clinical issues. Recent examples include research and development, recruitment and retention, and nurse prescribing.

The clinical governance imperative has presented opportunities for me to ensure that clinical matters are at the heart of the agenda of our trust board meetings. This is good news for nursing. The meetings are open meetings and thus nursing gains high profile with the public. The press recently gave coverage to a report I completed on bank nursing. Although the subsequent media coverage was not entirely pleasurable, the board paper made managers throughout the trust take the issue of bank and agency nursing seriously – not just because of costs but because it is a quality issue for our nursing staff in relation to continuity of patient care. Such papers would never have received an airing at board level in the business-orientated era of the NHS.

As a trust board we were required to set up a clinical governance committee and regular reports are also received by this committee, chaired by a non-executive trustee, on issues like clinical risk, quality of services and progress in encouraging clinical audit and research. There is regular analysis of complaints (and lessons learned) and routine examination of incidents, accidents and untoward events (e.g. suicides). The latter is done in the spirit of a 'learning organisation' with a concerted effort being made not to allocate blame but to learn lessons from failures and mistakes.

A good example of this in nursing, within the trust, is how we deal with 'medication errors'. In 1998 we introduced a 'medication error reporting' scheme. Details of this scheme were announced through our 'Safe Administration of Medicines' policy document, and the chief pharmacist and I publicised this at 'road shows' throughout the different sites within our trust. We encourage the reporting of medication errors and the scheme has been promoted as an equitable non-blame method of identifying clinical risk in relation to drug mistakes. Each individual report is confidentially and systematically collated, then analysed by a review team (consisting of the medical and nursing directors, the chief pharmacist and head of personnel). The specific professional groups get feedback on methods to minimise the risk of the error recurring.

To date, the reporting scheme has been successful in generating data for trend analysis, and there has been comparison, year on year of these data. We have been able to highlight where the incidence of errors has increased (e.g. wrong time of administration, drug omissions, controlled drugs, prescribing) and identified areas where the incidence of errors was reducing (e.g. vaccination, diabetic, self-medication). Through the reporting scheme we identify targets for improvement and direct the various professional groups to appropriate policies, procedures and guidelines. We have also developed and improved particular policies and developed competency-checking procedures. Although we strongly suspect that there is under-reporting of errors, as the number of errors has not increased in line with the expanded trust structures, we will continue to encourage use of the scheme as we believe that this systematic mechanism drives forward improvements in patient care. The system is not just for use by nurses but also identifies medication errors by pharmacists and doctors. This sort of system is supported in recent publications (*British Medical Journal*, 2000; Alberti, 2001).

The medical and nursing directors and the chief executive are called to account (at the clinical governance committee and its various sub-committees) for various trends in activity or patterns in practice. Although one is tempted to be defensive and recoil from such scrutiny, we are all beginning truly to engage in the work to measure our performance and work towards achieving 'best value', 'efficiency' and 'effectiveness'.

Clinical governance structures as a vehicle for change

We have established a clinical effectiveness group, chaired by an associate medical director, to give strategic leadership and a focus for clinical effectiveness activity in the trust. A sub-group has been established to take forward issues relating to the development and implementation of clinical guidelines. We also have a group looking at strategy, priorities and management issues surrounding audit. We have created audit structures relating to the independent contractors (GPs, dental practitioners, community pharmacist and practice nurses) and over time the work of these groups has become integrated and areas of activity extend across the quality spectrum.

Issue of clinical guidelines is essential to support clinical practice, and initially we set up a group to create an effective system for dissemination of guidelines, called Scottish Intercollegiate Guidelines Network (SIGN). Recently, we have launched the Lothian guidelines for 'hypertension' and 'management of patients with type 2 diabetes', developed two new guidelines, for 'lithium' and 'radiology', and updated the 'management of blood lipid disorders'. Our 'Lothian Joint Formulary' was also launched. This provides consistent advice on prescribing across all sectors and links to advice provided by the drug evaluation panel, a sub-committee of the area drug and therapeutic committee. Clearly there are costs associated with the dissemination and production of guidelines. Guidelines support evidence-based practice and clearly use of these lessens the chances of our staff giving poor patient care.

A good example of how guidelines can help promote good nursing practice is the implementation of the RCN and Department of Health-produced guidelines on depot neuroleptic injections (RCN/Department of Health, 1994). Standards within this document state that nurses should give information to patients, obtain user consent and assess the side effects of the medication. Additionally, good practice should entail nurses carrying out 'psychosocial interventions' with patients. These guidelines were issued to Community Psychiatric Nurses (CPNs) through their local nurse managers but in order to assess compliance with the standards, audits had to be done. The first was undertaken as part of a national audit (Pollock & Turner, 1998), and the second audit process was undertaken as part of the Clinical Standards Board Scotland (CSBS) visit, to assess compliance with the CSBS standards on schizophrenia (CSBS, 2001).

Both audits demonstrated good practice within our trust nursing staff, but the audit findings also demonstrated where nursing practice had to be improved. Following the former audit, the CPNs had to be trained to use systematic side-effect assessment tools, and following the CSBS visit there has been a concerted effort to train our mental health nurses in cognitive behaviour therapy. The latter was happening in fact, but the results of the audit, which were the substance of a written report, gave impetus to the speeding up of this training.

This example from mental health, then, provides an illustration that audit and implementation of guidelines is important. Again we see too, that it takes time for good guidelines to be used and truly put in practice.

Clinical governance and people governance

In our trust, we invest in the training and development of our staff. We are trying to create a culture of lifelong learning for our staff and support ongoing updating. We have an organisational learning, development and training function with three main components: organisational development and training department, the professional development unit and a general practice staff training team. Combined, these provide an increasingly integrated service in support of organisational, team and individual effectiveness. A training directory provides a list of in-house training programmes available to all staff. Training is provided in relation to all strands of clinical governance, e.g. research and development, clinical effectiveness, risk management, complaints and public involvement.

Specifically in relation to nursing, the clinical governance agenda has made it possible for me to lead in the development of a trust 'Nursing Policy and Protocols Manual' for all our trust nursing staff. This, in fact, was a major task. Initially a definition of 'policy' and 'protocol' had to be agreed and a framework and checklist devised for the development of these.

Prior to gaining such consensus, local teams were developing local policies and protocols, and, partly because several organisations merged, some staff were using inherited but out-of-date policies/protocols. This was unsatisfactory. There was duplication of effort in the trust, and lots of 're-invention' of wheels. Importantly too, this meant that different nurses in different parts of the trust were following 'local' policies and protocols. Thus, there was a variety of standards of nursing practice in place within the trust and time was being wasted, with the best of intentions, with groups of nurses trying to be accountable for their local practice.

There was a need to identify what policies needed to be standardised for trust-wide use, and an imperative to ensure that such policies/protocols were influenced by current research, evidence-based practice, clinical guidelines, UKCC/NMC directives and Government and national policies. Initial prioritisation resulted in the first issue of the manual containing clinical development policies (relating to the extended role of the nurse), tissue viability, palliative care and care of the dying and bereaved. Further work on child protection, continence management and infection control has taken place more recently, and an additional section of professional matters is to be added to the manual. Each policy/protocol has a review date and plans are in place to audit implementation of them. Crucially important, and a very good reason for developing the nursing manual, is that we could not develop clinical training programmes until the policies/protocols were completed. How could the clinical trainers decide what was to be included in the professional training for clinical competencies unless standards were clear?

Other key developments in people governance to support clinical governance include:

- the production of comprehensive guidelines for personal development planning and review, to support trust-wide appraisal
- the production of a trust policy for continuing personal development (CPD)
- the development and implementation of a targeted induction programme for nursing staff, mandatory training options

- the development of a competency framework for G-grade nursing staff and a G-grade development programme

These are developed in collaboration with staff representatives and supported by managers who release their staff on appropriate courses/training programmes. All these courses help ensure that staff have the skills to be competent in their jobs.

Clinical governance and its impact on nursing

The Royal College of Nursing (2000) illustrated how and why nurses should get involved in action to promote clinical governance. The development of clinical governance systems directly affects nurses as a major professional grouping within trusts. It is easy to quote anecdotal evidence that clinical governance is impacting positively on nurses. Examples that come to mind are that nurses in my trust are asking for training/appraisals/clinical supervision, asking for evidence-based policies to be developed in certain areas of practice, and demanding protected time to undertake audit (and research). None of this would have happened ten or even five years ago. In the past, nurses worked for years without appraisals, and were 'sent' on training. Policy manuals gathered dust on shelves and audit and research were anticipated with dread. I am not saying everything in the garden is rosy but we are seeing improvements in the desired direction.

But what evidence is there to demonstrate that the clinical governance environment is really impacting on nurses? As part of work to develop a 'Research and Development Strategy for Nursing in Scotland' a scoping exercise was done. Via questionnaires to nursing directors and heads of nursing departments, the intention was to ascertain progress made within trusts and HEIs to develop nurses to undertake research, or to develop nurses to become more research-orientated in their practice. The findings are fascinating (Hanley, 2002), and show that research and development is beginning to become a reality for nurses/nursing. Four of the 29 trusts who responded to the questionnaires stated that nurses had 'easy or very easy' access to libraries, and electronic libraries were recognised as a great improvement. IT support is still difficult and patchily developed in different trusts; some trusts did not have access to a librarian and some complained that their libraries had limited nursing resources.

Dissemination of research information is also being encouraged. Only two trusts had no method of distribution; and circulation was undertaken via newsletter, research interest groups, research days and web sites. One of the respondents said 'clinical governance activity, like audit and implementation of clinical guidelines, is raising nursing awareness of the application of research to care and helping to make nurses want to generate research'. This is surely proof – if proof is needed – that the clinical governance agenda is supporting nurses to be evidence-based practitioners.

The feedback from the surveys confirmed too, that a research culture is beginning to pervade nursing. A variety of initiatives are in place throughout trusts which support research endeavour (research fellowships, pilot funding, one month sabbaticals, in-house training for research, protected time for research-trained staff to 'do' research and the creation of nurse consultant posts). Some trusts had dedicated support for nurses to write research proposals and 25 of the 29 trusts said that they wanted help for their nurses to develop such proposals.

An environment of collaboration between the NHS and higher education institutions (HEIs) is also crucial as regards development of research and an evidence base (for nursing). The questionnaires confirmed that 11 of the 12 HEIs in Scotland had direct collaboration with NHS trusts on specific studies, or NHS personnel as co-grantholders. The NHS were permitting access to academic nurses for research studies and the latter in turn were helping novice researchers develop their ideas and seek funding. Historically, there has been an 'uneasy alliance' between academia and the health service, with the former having an 'ivory tower' image and being viewed by practitioners as remote and out of touch. That this is clearly not the situation today is due in no small measure to the policy imperatives enshrined in clinical governance. The latter is making the research process a legitimate activity for both academics and practitioners. Not all nurses want to or indeed are able to do research, but more and more nurses and all senior nurses are seeking research evidence to support their daily practice and wanting to follow protocols that are similarly rooted in an evidence base.

Nurses themselves know that they are accountable for their own practice. Such accountability has been evident historically in the professional guidance material sent, over the years, from the UKCC. It is even more evident in the latest *Code of Professional Conduct* (2002b), sent by the Nursing and Midwifery Council (the successor regulating body for nursing). I have no doubt that clinical governance activity is helping nurses, in a variety of ways, to be actually accountable for their practice, answerable for their actions and omissions, and to carry out a 'duty of care' to their patients and clients.

Clinical governance and cultural change

The assumption behind the introduction of clinical governance systems was that once they were in place we would move from being reactive and crisis-orientated, to being part of a culture in which we more proactively shape a health service based on primary prevention and achieve high quality healthcare everywhere.

Development towards high quality healthcare culture can be conceptualised as occurring in stages. I find this well illustrated by a model of 'stages of transition', the source of which I cannot locate. In the first stage, 'champions' (what were referred to in another context as 'hero innovators'), few in number, try to initiate change to improve the quality of healthcare. Over time, the numbers of those seeking to improve quality of care increases, but a significant difference occurs when all efforts to make improvements are fully concerted. Finally, through one means or another the efforts by all to improve healthcare quality become fully and predictably sustainable. We have gradually moved, over the past five years, through these stages towards becoming a 'high quality healthcare' organisation. I believe that we have moved from having few 'champions' of higher quality healthcare, to the present situation in which all our trust nurses are trying to make improvements, and some departments and teams may have reached the stage where collective efforts can be predictably sustained. I also firmly believe that clinical governance has helped our endeavours, and helped give our nurses direction and a sense of common purpose.

Confirmation that we are moving towards sustainable work towards improving the quality of healthcare is readily available in our trust. Clinical governance activity is no longer purely top-down driven. It is bottom-up driven and top-down supported. We have a clinical governance support team that helps services undertake audits. Field staff themselves are striving to take a more systematic approach to their daily work. Validated screening tools are being used and assessed for efficacy; outcome measures are being developed for application, and services/practice/procedures are being evaluated. We have moved from striving for accreditation awards (e.g. Chartermark) as a 'must do', to departments and GP practices taking an active role in developing national accreditation systems and volunteering to take part in internal peer review systems to support continuous quality improvements. Nursing is crucially involved in all of this work – testimony, I believe, that nurses want to be accountable for their practice and really find out if they are doing the best they possibly can for patients.

Sharing good practice

We try very hard within our trust to encourage staff to share and generalise good practice. Obviously this saves time and avoids duplication of effort. From the management perspective we do not want staff wasting time repeating work that has already been undertaken elsewhere in the trust. We hold various events to try and share good practice, via conferences and quality days with a series of oral presentations and poster displays. Some of these have multidisciplinary attendance with a wide range of professions and services represented, other occasions are uni-disciplinary in terms of focus, e.g. the Annual Nursing Conference, with a varied audience. We have a clinical governance newsletter that enables sharing of ideas and good practice across the trust and it also provides a stimulus for staff to undertake further pieces of work to enhance patient care.

Sharing of good practice, however, is hard work as we continually come across the necessary ingredient of change – ownership. Many areas do not want to just adopt someone else's work, they want to tinker with it and 'make it their own'. We also find that many areas are reluctant to share their good work, because they are not used to 'blowing their own trumpet'. We have not found the answer to this problem but we are sure that we must keep on with our attempts at sharing and dissemination. With time this may get easier – not just for nursing but for all staff groups.

Evidence-based practice – the reality

There are very real problems, from the management perspective, about putting evidence-based practice into place. Circulation of evidence-based guidelines alone is insufficient to ensure that the guidelines are being followed. Time needs to be spent consulting/debating/discussing them with the various stakeholders, and up-to-date guidance needs to be part of the training for staff. Key staff also need to be convinced of the merits of evidence-based practice. Old habits die hard! Our experience has been that individual teams and groups of nurses (and other staff) want to customise tools that have been validated and proven to be reliable (by traditional research methods), thus negating the previous research work. We have also found that implementation of evidence-based guidelines is costly, not only in terms of time invested by senior staff, but also in relation to real financial costs (of purchasing and using copyrighted assessment tools, for instance). Undoubtedly, though, it is worth persevering, as the benefits of changing practice and promoting high quality care outweigh the disadvantages of complaints, poor care and, at worst, defending a litigation case.

In summary, developing clinical governance systems cannot be done overnight. Management and 'quality' gurus say it takes between eight and twelve years to change a culture. I am sure it will take us at least that to change the culture within nursing from being reactive to proactive. Traditionally the Health Service has not invested adequately in its nurses in terms of staff development, and it certainly has not invested sufficiently in promoting a research culture or in systems to prevent accidents, errors and mistakes. But this situation is changing and the climate of clinical governance has been a major driver of attitude change.

Clinical governance is a major influencing factor, too, in terms of helping managers develop credible systems for which they can be called to account. These managers (and I hope I am one of them) are increasingly seen by staff to be directly supporting them in their roles – for which they in turn, are accountable. Walshe (1998a, b) suggests that to implement clinical governance three elements will be required: accountability for clinical performance; internal trust mechanisms for improving performance; and external mechanisms for improving clinical performance. If not in place, clinical governance will be nothing more than words. I can conclude by saying I believe that in Scotland, and most definitely here in my Trust, for nursing the rhetoric is being turned into reality.

Chapter 9

Working with Children: Accountability and Paediatric Nursing

Gosia Brykczyñska

Introduction

At an extraordinary session of the UN, the children of the world prepared a statement concerning their ongoing desires and rights for the special session on children, held at the beginning of May 2002. Among several rights and issues commented upon they elaborated upon their right to adequate and appropriate healthcare and the need for the world to address the issues of HIV/AIDS in young people. They requested that they have 'affordable and accessible life-saving drugs and treatment . . . and strong and accountable partnerships established among all to promote better health for children' (UNICEF, 2002). Moreover, nurses are also constantly being told by their regulatory bodies that they are responsible and, above all, accountable for their professional practice to the public (Clark, 2000).

It is less clear, however, what is meant by the words 'responsible' or 'accountable'. Styles (1985), in an interesting article on the nature of accountability, rightly points out that 'as a word gains popularity it loses clarity. Accountability is one such endangered word.' Not only is the word not clearly understood by those who would appear to be most obviously affected by it but, depending on the professional and/or vocational outlook of the user of the word, it may take on quite varying and specific connotations. Thus, for modern healthcare workers accountability has about it an inevitable ring of testimony and reporting – a rather defensive reaction to some past event; a reporting back of junior to senior professional. Philosophers, however, see accountability mainly through the prism of its chief constituent or, as Bergman (1981) noted, its 'key component', which is, responsibility.

This chapter will provide an analysis of accountability in relation to paediatric nursing and children, presenting first some definitions of paediatric nursing and then of children, in order to set the context for a review of accountability based on Bergman's schema for nursing accountability. Bergman, in analysing the dimensions of accountability, saw the need for a necessary hierarchical infrastructure to be in place in order for true professional accountability to be possible. Thus, what Bergman refers to as ability, that is, skills and values, philosophers refer to rather more globally as knowledge, particularly personal knowledge – or as Russell (1991) said, 'knowledge by acquaintance'.

Moreover, most healthcare professionals tend to talk of the necessity for the presence of an 'authority' to act, that is, an authority which is vested in the moral agent by virtue of rank, education, charisma and/or legal power. To have authority implies, therefore, the presence of a freedom to act autonomously in particular situations, and the freedom to be able to delegate justifiably. There is no real authority unless one has the freedom to manoeuvre, freedom to choose certain acts and freedom to go down certain paths (Glover, 1970; Nuttall, 1993). It is only when ability and authority are adequately matched that one can start analysing the true nature of responsibility, which in turn contributes to the profession's understanding of accountability for practice.

Definition of paediatric nursing

Paediatric nurses have a wide remit. Paediatric nursing is a special branch of professional nursing requiring specific knowledge and skills concerning the health and welfare of children. Within this one can specialise even further, for example in oncology nursing, community nursing, school nursing and intensive care. Meanwhile, the scope of practice of children's nurses is changing fast. Currently there is a need to re-evaluate the traditional terms and understanding of paediatric nursing accountability. Not only do the nurses care for the sick child in traditional hospital settings, they also care for seriously ill children in the home, in paediatric hospices and on psychiatric units. Additionally, they take under their wings healthy children and chronically ill children who are living in the community and work with them and their families in order to maintain their health, in schools, clinics and outpatient departments. In fact, paediatric nurses are concerned with the health and wellbeing of the whole child, wherever the child or youngster may be (Glasper & Tucker, 1993). Therefore it can be said that paediatric nurses are focused on the health and welfare of the whole child, from neonate to adolescent.

Describing the patient group which is the focus of paediatric nursing is complex. Notions of childhood, according to some historians, are relatively recent, and indeed in some parts of the world an individual over the age of six or seven is accorded a place in society akin to that reserved for adults elsewhere (James & Prout, 1990; Archard, 1993). Children are considered to be smaller versions of adults, and have to compete with them for natural resources and contribute very early in their life to the economic wellbeing of their society. The children are often exploited and abused. In such societies there rarely exists the notion of adolescence as we know it. This point has been eloquently demonstrated in the Amnesty International document (1995) *Childhood Stolen*, and in a rather shocking article by Fasting and her Danish nurse colleagues on the illegal trade of children's body parts (Fasting *et al.*, 1998). This has been reiterated and confirmed more recently by the children of the world themselves at the extraordinary meeting of the UN, The United Nations Special Session on Children in New York in May 2002.

It appears that the adult world is not listening to children, in spite of the fact that the rights of a child to be taken seriously and listened to are clearly enshrined in the UN Convention of Children's Rights (1989) adopted by HM Government in 1991. The adult world is not taking on board the full weight of their responsibilities regarding children. In contemporary European and industrial settings, it is societal demands placed upon nurses working with children and their families which help to shape and orient nurses' own understanding of their professional accountability regarding young people and children. Additionally, unlike nurses working with adults, the nurses must always bear in mind the collaborative and, in some cases, co-opted caring role which they play alongside that of parents and legally defined primary carers.

Accountability, in the context of paediatric nursing, is not just a question of moral responsibility for one's personal or even collective actions. It is also always, simultaneously, an expression of facilitation and empowerment of the families and the children themselves to a level of accountability and readiness to share in the responsibilities of health maintenance, health promotion and the restoration of health. Precisely because children are not held fully responsible for their actions, adults who come into contact with children must start to initiate them into the necessity for increasing their levels of responsibility for particular actions and decisions. Accountability for healthcare decisions in a paediatric context, if it is to be truly patient centred, must also always be a form of collective responsibility between various professional groups, the family, the child and society, where the children themselves outline the framework within which accountability can and must be discussed.

Ability

In order to be held accountable for actions and decisions, one needs to be capable of discerning morally correct acts and be competent to undertake moral and social decisions and be appropriately prepared to do so. Several contemporary philosophers have discussed the possible reasoning which lay behind Aristotle's strong condemnation of those individuals who make incorrect moral choices, even if those choices were made under duress (Aristotle, 1962; Lloyd, 1969). Aristotle differentiated between the universal moral knowledge that one ought to have (and should be striving to continually expand and cultivate), and specific knowledge, which might legitimately be missing. The general universal knowledge of right and wrong is so fundamental to the nature of the mature moral agent that there is little one can say by way of excuse to mitigate a wrong choice or act.

Likewise, in paediatric nursing there is a body of knowledge which is considered 'universal', and all qualified paediatric nurses are expected to be familiar with these facts and observations. All children's nurses must know the difference between a normal neonatal heart rate and that of a toddler's, or the levels of expected social development in an eight-year-old and an adolescent. What an outsider would consider specific knowledge is considered routine and basic for someone working within the field of paediatrics. However, the knowledge and competencies which are required of the professionals form part of the accepted universal backdrop against which their professional decisions can and should be made, and against which the paediatric nurse can be held accountable. Should a paediatric nurse not know or be unfamiliar with part of this canon of paediatric nursing practice, by that same deficiency they would be declaring themselves outside the body of professional paediatric nursing.

This point was well emphasised in the recommendations following the publication of the Clothier Report (1994), which were presented to the public after the inquiry investigating the devastating acts perpetrated by Miss Beverley Allitt in 1991. The entire healthcare team, from the school of nursing through hospital managers and paediatric consultants, down to the staff nurses, were held accountable for not taking adequate responsibility for the routine work that they were doing. The paediatric team, in particular, was held accountable for not appreciating the significance of a string of most unusual deaths and incidents which occurred during a short space of time on the children's ward. One such untoward event would have been most unusual but several such events was definitely beyond the norm for paediatrics and called for drastic action and a moratorium on patient admissions.

The local consultant paediatrician insisted upon a paediatric post-mortem to be performed by a paediatric pathologist on one of Beverley Allitt's victims, since he was profoundly disturbed by the unexpected death of the child. This was an unusual death and needed to be investigated by a specialist. However, the doctor's request, based upon his expertise of children, was ignored in large measure because of the additional cost that this request would entail and because the general managers and non-specialist pathologists did not appreciate what the consultant paediatrician was telling them. As the report concluded, specialist services should be engaged 'in every case in which the death of a child is unexpected or clinically unaccountable'.

One can always be wise with hindsight, and it can now be seen that the deaths caused by Beverley Allitt were most unusual and not entirely preventable. However, much could and should have been done that would have minimised her access to children and therefore the damage which she could do, and much more could have been done to listen to the opinion of the local paediatric specialists who knew that something most peculiar was occurring. The paediatric staff nurses working alongside her were also held accountable for not appreciating the true significance of the children's deaths and near misses, and for tolerating low standards of practice, such as low levels of qualified paediatric staff working on the unit. It is sad to think that almost ten years later the Bristol Inquiry (Secretary of State, 2001) still saw fit to comment that: 'All healthcare staff who treat children must have training in caring for children.'

In summary, in order to be held professionally accountable one must have at least a minimum level of competency and skill relevant to that profession or discipline. Aristotle, referring to Greek citizens, expected a basic universal level of moral discernment in order for individuals to be held morally responsible. In the same way, in the example of specialised professional practice, there is a specific body of knowledge that one must possess in order to be able to practise one's art. The possession of this specific professional knowledge carries with it certain obligations.

Obligations

One of the many obligations which may follow increased awareness concerning the knowledge of a child's psychosocial and physical development may be the need for a certain measure of political activism, in order to ensure that children in our society receive and are aware of their minimum human rights. This type of social and professional awareness may therefore involve lobbying local councils and health authorities for better facilities for children. Alternatively, it may also mean the need for closer liaison with other childcare workers, for example playleaders and nursery schoolteachers. Certainly, awareness of the needs of children and youngsters does not and should not finish with the completion of an eight-hour shift. It should form part of one's total value system and, therefore, be fundamental to our understanding of child welfare and most significantly, influence our ethical and professional and personal decision-making processes.

Unfortunately, we are made most aware of lapses in this area when something goes seriously wrong, such as the lack of follow-up and communication among childcare workers as evidenced during the brief life of Victoria Climbie. Victoria was a young girl who was physically and mentally abused by her relatives, and an inquiry concluded that, despite having been admitted and treated for injuries several times on a paediatric unit, paediatricians and paediatric nurses did not adequately follow up her care (The Victoria Climbie Inquiry: www.victoria-climbie-inquiry.org.uk).

One of the obligations that befalls paediatric healthcare workers is the duty to communicate with the entire healthcare and social work team about problematic cases, even after the strictly medical side of concerns is taken care of. Children are by definition vulnerable members of society, not always in a position to speak up for themselves, and unfortunately their parents or guardians do not always care properly for them. Better communication among the childcare team members who are alerted to potential problems would go a long way to solving some of these complications and preventing tragedies from occurring.

Such high levels of knowledge about ill children, and a commitment to children and adolescents in the community and society at large, do not come vicariously. It falls upon professional paediatric nurse lecturers to inculcate the next generation of nurses, not only with the crucial level of paediatric values which will form the moral core of paediatric nursing, but also the necessary levels of appreciation for the paediatric arts and sciences. As Cook (1990) observed:

> If nursing education is the core of the profession, the nurse educationalists have a responsibility to the practitioner, the helper and the manager, since they must, to some extent, provide the knowledge and skills for professionals to become accountable.

That nurses need a certain level of competence in order to be held accountable for creative, positive practice seems reasonable, but what about the parents who share in the child's care?

Involving parents

Modern paediatric nursing is practised together with a child's parents, and accountability for paediatric practice includes the concept of collective accountability of all those working with a child – not only qualified professionals. Since the most important beings in the life of a child are the child's parents, and it is they who predominantly care for the child, it is also they who bear the greatest share of moral and social responsibility for the welfare of the child. The relevant question, therefore, is what level of expertise and ability can be expected of parents in order for them to be considered accountable, together with the nurse, for the care of a child? This question has been posed and investigated by several sociologists and legal experts who have concluded that parents, like anyone else, need to be informed about their children's welfare in order to be fully competent to make meaningful consents to treatment on behalf of their children. With older children the children themselves need to be consulted together with the parents (Alderson, 1996; Alderson, 2000).

The educative role of nurses is well documented. It starts with educative antenatal classes, where prospective parents are helped and guided, as necessary and appropriate, by various members of the professional nursing team right through the child's infancy and childhood. Parents of the chronically ill child however, may quickly outstrip professionals in specific knowledge of their child. This is certainly the case as regards specific habits, social customs, preferences and even information where physiological norms are concerned. The educative role of the professional in such circumstances is, literally, to fill in the gaps, in order for the parents to make a more coherent picture of the whole that will enable them to continue caring for and being responsible for their own child. It is all the more interesting, therefore, that many professionals in the healthcare field still regard parents' knowledge and abilities with considerable suspicion. Alderson (1990), in her landmark book *Choosing for Children*, which concerns parental informed consent for children, superbly documents the attitude of some surgeons to the decision-making capacities of parents. Thus she records one consultant as saying:

> Don't expect much of parents. Some are good witnesses and some are vague and not terribly helpful. In episodic events I may rely on them, but I tell them what is likely to happen, that the child may become blue. . . . It's a way of handling it and involving parents. I don't rely on their opinion. I prefer to go on objective clinical data.   (Alderson, 1990)

Obviously the surgeon is clinically responsible for performing the right operation at the right time, but it is the parents who have to agree to the surgery and it is they who are accountable to society for caring for their child and providing, by consent, adequate medical care. The incompetence of some cardiac surgeons which recently came to light at the Bristol Royal Infirmary (BRI) reminds us of the inordinate pressures which parents feel when making decisions for their children concerning life-saving treatments and interventions. Although the paediatric team is responsible for maintaining a high level of competence, and the Bristol Inquiry upheld this position very clearly, the parents also feel emotionally and morally responsible for the care of their child. It is they who have to agree to surgery and they feel violated and let down when it transpires that there is a cloak of secrecy and conspiracy regarding poor work practices and incompetence that affects the care and outcomes of their children's admission to hospital (Secretary of State, 2001). As the inquiry noted: 'there must be openness about clinical performance. Patients should be able to gain access to information about the relative performance of a hospital.'

The level of parental accountability for making correct decisions, and appropriately caring for their child, is immeasurably increased and augmented by the intervention and cooperation, if not the advocacy, of paediatric nurses. This truism is most clearly demonstrated when it is absent. The parent who refuses reasonable treatment for a child is an obvious example. Even more startling are the instances where nurses agree with parents about decisions not to treat a child for an otherwise treatable disorder or symptom. It is of course the case that often it is not clear what clinical decisions should be made in the child's best interest, and not only does the welfare of an individual child come into play but also aspects of the parents' religion and culture. Accountability of parents for their children's welfare, however, is of paramount legal, social and emotional importance. Moreover, in law, parental participation in the consenting process is considered to be a responsibility rather than a right.

This observation was upheld by the High Court in the Gillick case. In that case, Lord Scarman told Mrs Gillick that, in effect, she had parental rights over her children only as long as she also fulfilled her parental responsibilities (i.e. those of parenting) and was actively involved in parenting her children (Dyer, 1985). The fundamental task of paediatric nurses is to work with parents so that they can continue actively parenting their child throughout the child's illness, and to be in a reasonable position to be accountable for the care given to their child. In many respects modern paediatric nursing is care delivered by proxy. Accountability is, therefore, also referred out to parents to the extent that parents have been given the necessary skills and competence to do so by paediatric nurses and the entire childcare team (Alderson, 1990).

Autonomy of children

If paediatric nurses share with parents the accountability for a young patient's welfare, what personal decision-making skills and aptitudes are required of the child for the child to be considered as an autonomous, competent moral agent? Certainly some children, as with some adults, can be held accountable for cooperation with the healthcare team (Alderson, 1993). Thus, even fairly young children with spina bifida can be taught how to self-catheterize and look after their basic needs, only reporting back and consulting with the school or paediatric community nurse as and when appropriate. It is no longer the responsibility of the parent or the nurse to ensure continence once the child or youngster has learnt the requisite skills and is deemed competent to function independently at school. Competent children take over responsibility for that area of their life. Good nursing accountability, however, demands that the child knows it can have access to a school or community nurse, and that the nurse is aware of the child's progress and is concerned with liaising between the child, the parents, the school and the referral centre.

Children who have chronic illnesses, for example diabetes or asthma, can also be held accountable for self-medication and, in cooperation with the school nurse, take on essentially adult healthcare responsibilities as and when appropriate. In such an instance, a nurse, or a member of the community child health team is held accountable for ensuring that such children and their parents are given the necessary guidance; that there is access to emergency care; and that relevant adults, such as teachers, know how to intervene appropriately, and so on. In all these cases children are slowly introduced to the world of adult responsibilities as far as their healthcare needs are concerned, for such an approach truly respects children as individuals who are capable, when appropriately prepared, to take on such responsibilities in respect of their competencies (Alderson, 1993).

There is a natural tendency to shield ill people from a bad prognosis, or an uncertain diagnosis, leading to the natural conclusion that they should not participate actively in decision-making about their treatment. Some paediatricians even discourage active cooperation by children with their relatively routine treatment protocols, and the young patient is expected to be entirely passive. There is however, a paradox here: in order to make a positive difference to health outcomes, one needs to be involved in the treatment plans, that is, be aware of one's diagnosis and agree to treatment plans. This truism is as relevant for children as it is for adults, and the agreement and cooperation of parents alone is not sufficient for even small children once past the toddler stage and certainly not for older children, youngsters and adolescents. Again it is one of the recommendations of the Bristol Inquiry that all staff working with children 'be trained in communicating with young people and parents' (Secretary of State, 2001).

Few examples of the burden of emotional labour experienced by nurses is as painfully obvious as when having to tell patients that they are not likely to survive their illness. In the context of paediatric nursing the question arises as to who takes on this responsibility, and to what extent children should know that they are dying. Can one actually be ethically accountable for imparting such information to a child? Children, as much as adults, like to be in control of their lives and their own affairs. To the extent that they are capable of this they are likewise accountable to their family and society for their brief lives. As one mother recounted, she imparted to her adolescent son the information about his impending death with a certain amount of trepidation, albeit with far more authority and love than any professional paediatric worker ever could. Thus she said:

> Two or so days before he died, I manoeuvered separate conversations with both our children that imparted that knowledge to them. Hamish reacted not with fear or horror, but as if he had just been told he should go for a walk on a very stormy day – 'Mama, I'd really rather not.'
> (Cooper & Harpin, 1991)

Responsibility for imparting important information to children should normally lie with the parents, who will obviously need support and help from professionals. In keeping with the entire ethos of modern child-centred paediatric care, it is hard to envisage treating a child who does not know his or her diagnosis (Alderson, 1990, 1993). Paediatric nurses' accountability lies in supporting the parents in this role of imparting information to children – and only when the parents cannot perform this task should they intervene (Casey, 1993). Assessment of the parents' competence to take over this hitherto traditionally professional task lies within the remit of good paediatric nursing and medicine.

Authority

It has often been said that there can be no accountability for practice where there is no true autonomy of action. If actions are performed under undue duress, or tasks omitted because of lack of choice, then moral philosophers would start to question the level of freedom and free will a person is experiencing. We can only be accountable for that over which we as individuals exercise a degree of authority (Glover, 1970; French, 1993). Additionally, authority, in the context of paediatric nursing, can be either the nurses' personal authority over their own actions, stemming at least in part from expertise and in part from invested hierarchical structures; or authority that a nurse vests in the parents, who are the child's main caregivers.

Thus, as with competence, it is not only the nurse's authority that is being discussed but also the patient's and the family's. The nurse, in truth, has no authority to act for or with a child except that granted to them by the parents and, increasingly, by the child (HM Government, 1989, 1991; Tingle, 1991; Alderson, 1993). This shift in the focus of authority, and therefore in moral perspective, is extremely important. It is not the nurses' authority and level of free will over their own actions that is solely at stake, but the level of autonomy and authority the young patients and their families have over their actions that are of paramount importance in paediatric nursing (Alderson, 1993).

Free will and choice

Issues of free will are central, therefore, to arguments about moral behaviour. Without sufficient free will there can be no discussion about moral choices. If mature individuals are to be responsible for their actions they must be able to choose those behaviours and to act in those ways that support particular moral intentions (Glover, 1970; Nuttall, 1993). Nurses often say that they would like to behave in a certain way, to conduct themselves in a particular fashion, but feel that they do not have the freedom or authority to do so. It is difficult to talk of accountability for practice if there is no corresponding authority of action to match the level of competency and insight (Lanara, 1982).

Aristotle, in his *Nicomachean Ethics*, was not particularly lenient with people who stated that they behaved against their better judgement even under duress. He felt that it was important to structure one's life in such a way as to be more in control more of the time and that unpleasantness may be an inevitable consequence of making an ethical decision; that is, some morally correct judgements may be unpleasant or difficult to make. Often we complain about lack of authority to act in the way we would like to, when in reality we have not done all that we could to structure our environment to be more conducive to a particular ethical milieu (Aristotle, 1962; Lanara, 1982).

It has been increasingly clear for some time now, and particularly since the findings of the Bristol Inquiry that healthcare workers would like to point out defects in the system or would like to stop a bad practice from continuing but they are often bullied into silence, while whistle-blowers are actively ostracised and condemned (Hunt, 1998). The Inquiry, therefore, found that 'The culture of the future must be a culture of public service in which collaborative teamwork is prized; and a culture of flexibility in which innovation can flourish in response to patient's needs' (Secretary of State, 2001).

In the interest of patient safety, a more transparent NHS and public accountability there are now new laws in place governing whistle-blowing and the criminalisation of acts of bullying and other such activities. As the Bristol Inquiry noted:

> Incentives for reporting events should be introduced, whereby healthcare professionals' contracts would provide that they would be immune from disciplinary action from their employer or professional regulatory body if they were to report a sentinel event. . . . Confidential reporting should be provided for. Failure to report would attract possible disciplinary action.
>
> (Secretary of State, 2001)

These issues have been picked up and elaborated from the Whistle-blowing and the Public Interest Disclosure Act 1998. However, as Catherine Hobby (2001) points out, 'A potential whistle-blower should recognise that the act of whistle-blowing still has a negative image, despite the enactment of legal protection'. This is where professional and statutory bodies could play a greater role both in protecting the reporting professional and in helping to create a more open climate within the NHS and healthcare generally. As Hunt (1998) comments 'The whistle-blower shows us that this is a time when accountabilities are shifting, or can be shifted to encompass a wider arena of stakeholders.'

Power and political action

Perhaps one of the most stressful situations for the nursing profession is having the knowledge and skills to direct specific actions, but to feel deprived of the power to influence and promote the necessary change (Lanara, 1982; Styles, 1985). Paediatric nurses have long known that small children need to be nursed in purpose-designed paediatric specialty wards. Children fare better when looked after by their parents on wards catering for their specific needs. In spite of this accepted child-centred wisdom, there has been no legal power to back up these findings until some of the more recent Government recommendations and legal interventions.

However, in the short term, if a hospital or primary care trust (PCT) does not want to provide separate accident and emergency services for children, or separate ear, nose and throat specialty beds serviced by paediatric nurses, then paediatric nurses by themselves do not have the power to create these necessary changes. Such situations, where personal knowledge of professionally correct conduct clashes with management and economic realities, highlight the essential impotence that nurses often feel.

Paediatric nurses, however, are not altogether without influence and, together with parent interest groups, can and should lobby for particular changes. It is precisely as a result of these lobbying activities over many years that the Bristol Inquiry could say that there is a need for better paediatric services, and that there must be a a way of articulating a voice for children's healthcare (including even a national service framework for children), be-cause 'the healthcare needs of children are different from those of adults and this must be recognised' (Secretary of State, 2001).

Ultimately, power and authority comes to those who actively seek it. Consumer groups, such as Action for Sick Children (ASC), formerly the National Association for the Welfare of Children in Hospital (NAWCH), have developed an authority base over the past 25 years, which few modern governments would dare to ignore totally. Lobby groups may not have the last say, but in a democratic society they do represent the vested power of an otherwise voiceless group. ASC, together with the Paediatric Society of the Royal College of Nursing and the Royal College of Paediatrics and Child Health (RCPCH), have co-written several significant guidelines and advisory documents which clearly outline the philosophy and orientation of modern child-centred healthcare.

Eventually, governments will have to accommodate the recommendations of these expert specialist groups. The authority of modern paediatric nurses is not self-generated or self-serving. Rather, it stems from the concerted effort to be in tandem with parental thinking, other child-centred groups and, obvi-ously, the thinking and desires of the children themselves. The old adage that there is power (and authority) in numbers has much to recommend it. The central problem with all childcare services is that although children form roughly a quarter of the entire population they take up a considerably smaller percentage of the healthcare budget. In order for things to change in favour of children's services, much lobbying and work will still have to be done on behalf of children and youngsters. However, the tide is apparently changing in favour of children, even if it has taken events at the Bristol Royal Infirm-ary and the actions of Beverley Allitt to spearhead the necessity for change.

There is a constant political temptation to marginalise paediatric services and reduce the paediatric healthcare budget because, the argument goes, children cannot speak up for themselves and do not have the power to vote. Currently, the authority and power to positively influence child health-centred change comes, paradoxically, not from interested third parties – that is, paediatric healthcare workers and other members of society – but from the children and the parents themselves who are taking seriously the need to be responsible for their own healthcare needs and to obtain recognition of their rights. As long as the moral, legal and social authority to act in the realm of healthcare provisions was seen solely as the province of healthcare workers, the outcomes of the delivery of children's healthcare seemed rather predictable. The recommendations of the Secretary of State (2001) came none too soon for the safety and welfare of children in the UK, and possibly the single most important point which the inquiry made was the need for more open, transparent and responsive delivery of healthcare in relation to the health needs of children.

Now that parents and their children are demanding a greater share in the say about healthcare structures, and are voicing their own authoritative demands, it is impossible to foretell all the consequences of this approach and where this may lead us. Meanwhile, shared collective responsibility for healthcare provision should itself lower overall anxieties and concerns related to paediatric healthcare services. In this fashion, after much heartache and blundering, a creative collective approach to children's services is being arrived at by the healthcare professions in answer to the moral imperative to care for children, in partnership with the parents and the children and young people themselves (Alderson, 1990, 1993; Casey, 1993).

Responsibility

Much has been written about the importance of responsibility in connection with accountability. Nurses are encouraged to be responsible for their nursing actions, as conscious responsibility will contribute to overall higher levels of accountability. It is interesting that Lanara defines responsibility as being 'dependent upon knowledge, discretion, judgement, and the ability to make decisions about one's work'. She sees responsibility as something over which the informed, reflective nurse has considerable control. Philosophers, however, are not as uniformly sure about levels and the nature of responsibility. To be responsible implies being answerable, or accountable, either to another or oneself for some act or acts. Responsibility implies moral accountability for one's actions, a capability for rational conduct, and for fulfilling obligations for vested trust. It means justifying a trust; to be reliable. Such dictionary type definitions, however, obscure some of the more complex questions associated with the proposition.

As French (1993) comments, many people would hold that 'a person is morally responsible for what he has done only if he could have done otherwise'; a proposition not altogether foreign to the average moral agent working in a healthcare context. This sentiment presupposes two fundamental premises in the discourse concerning responsibility: first, that the moral agent is acting in good faith with free will – that is, is uncoerced; and second, that there is a known (or even unknown) choice of actions available. There is an emphasis in this particular presentation of professional responsibility on free will and choice, two moral ingredients not necessarily always present or in fact capable of being equally present. French calls this situation the principle of alternative possibilities (PAP), and PAP most evidently cannot always be honoured. Many professionally morally correct acts, resulting from a measure of responsibility, are undertaken in the knowledge of either no acceptable alternatives or, indeed, any other alternative, given a particular desired objective.

Responsibilities for treatment

Several years ago a health visitor, against universally accepted wisdom, encouraged a mother to discontinue taking her child to the oncology clinic.

The nurse was rightly held morally responsible for contributing to the untimely death of the child. She was held responsible even though she claimed she was working with the mother. The same could be said of a Jehovah's Witness parent whose child requires a blood transfusion, or the parent who refuses a treatment option on the basis of religious convictions, as in a recent case of the need to separate conjoined twins (Brykczyñska, 2000). The fact that the parent's religious or cultural convictions curtail the range of medical interventions which they may feel comfortable adopting does not absolve the parents from the moral responsibility of refusing particular treatments.

On the whole, physicians and healthcare workers do respect the rights of parents to make treatment decisions. As already noted it is the parent's right and responsibility to make these decisions. However, just occasionally, especially if there is an obvious conflict of interest over the consequences of the proposed treatment options, the resolution of the problem may have to be made by the courts, and always in favour of the best interests of the child principle. Certainly, such instances of apparent conflict of interest are a call for the healthcare system to be less complacent about its apparent superiority and to search diligently for alternative treatments and approaches which are more acceptable to the parents concerned and the general public. Finally, it is good to repeat the often quoted truism that in a moral context to do nothing is to choose to do something, and that 'something' is also a morally and legally binding choice.

Responsibility can also be seen as a form of liability, and it was almost presented this way by the surgeons concerned with the treatment of the Maltese conjoined twins, separated in Manchester in 2000 (Brykczyñska, 2000). For others, responsibility is seen as a bothersome consequence of morality which can curb overzealous righteousness, or it may prompt action where otherwise nothing would be happening. It can also be likened to a barter game, as French (1993) proposes, since 'we spend a considerable (perhaps inordinate) amount of time trying to avoid responsibility wherever and whenever possible'. The need to avoid responsibility and the act of passing it on to someone else stems from the logical deduction that responsibility involves accepting obligations and performing actions for which one can be held accountable. As French astutely observes 'no wonder that avoidance of responsibility has become almost an art form, one that is learned and practised relatively early in life and honed to the end'.

It is quite natural to strive to avoid responsibility, even if increased responsibility means considerably more kudos and economic remuneration. Paediatric nurses, traditionally, have not gone out of their way to court responsibility, but much is changing. With a new emphasis on the need for increased skills and hands-on therapeutic interventions, paediatric nurses are realising that there may be a correspondingly greater level of responsibility but also, more specifically, an increased level of work satisfaction. As French noted 'People merit praise and blame for what they do, and not just "on the basis" of what they do'.

Consequences of responsibility

Translating this into nursing language, we would say that paediatric nurses are found to be accountable and are deemed to be responsible (with corresponding praise or blame) in direct proportion to the extent to which they are seen to have behaved in praiseworthy or blameworthy fashion. It is not the profession of paediatric nursing, however, that is most often under scrutiny but the specific conduct of particular nurses. French (1993) claims that: 'the responsibility barter game (RBG) is probably the most common experience ordinary people have with morality'. This is because everyone, including nurses, aims to avoid and pass on all possible extraneous responsibility, in spite of any possible benefits (and there usually are some) that might ensue from increased obligations and accountability.

Few people are as aware of the ramifications of increased responsibilities as parents and healthcare workers and among them paediatric nurses. Nurses are also aware of the increased prestige and gratification that accompanies increased responsibility, due to extended role performance. Nonetheless, although it would seem that increased responsibility should be everyone's aim and ambition, increased levels of responsibility are a factor for individual negotiation rather than a foregone conclusion relevant to all professionals (or even parents) based on a decree from superior managers or family psychologists. As French observes, 'People's lives are affected when responsibility is ascribed, assessed and accepted'; it has profound moral implications for the actors in the game and, on balance, the less direct responsibility and the more indirect credit one has, the better one feels. No one wants to manage an understaffed paediatric intensive care unit, but nurses readily bask in the public praise heaped on 'heroic angels' fighting to save babies' lives. Ironically, it was just such thinking taken to its extreme form that triggered enrolled nurse Beverley Allitt into a psychiatric condition resulting in her killing spree in the spring of 1991.

Curiously, as French notes, too much praise is also to be avoided, perhaps because of the fickle nature of public opinion, and it is altogether seen to be more psychologically stable to avoid as much positive as negative publicity and comment. There is, of course, another, more deep-seated reason why discomfort arises in giving praise and blame for accepted responsibility. It is very difficult to be sure of the true motives behind someone's actions and, therefore, to judge whether an action for which we are responsible by virtue of our profession is to be regarded as praiseworthy and/or exceptional. The motive behind the action for it to be considered praiseworthy would need to be something above and beyond the call of duty and akin to a type of heroic altruism.

Some aspects of this observation have been investigated by nurse researchers such as Sarah Hutchinson in 1989, who followed up nurses who claimed to have broken regulations in order to be accountable to the patient, putting their nursing careers and professionalism in a difficult moral situation; or Kubsch (1996), who has investigated how autonomous decisions are made by nurses. However, few paediatric nurses can claim to work entirely from altruistic motives. Motives for moral actions are usually mixed and demonstrate, in the same person at any one time, varying degrees of moral and personal interest.

This line of research has been also been followed up by Hunt (1997) who echoes Hutchinson's earlier work saying, that occasionally under exceptional and mitigating circumstances, it may be necessary to break the rules of conduct or to break the rules of the establishment. He refers to the prevalence of 'occupational subordination'. How often do nurses dismiss praise (even routine praise) with the disclaimer 'Oh, that was nothing, I was doing my duty', or, 'That was nothing, anyone would have done likewise', even though these nurses have many years of professional training. They have often put much of themselves into the task at hand, and in truth, not everyone would have done what had just been performed. It is, therefore, not just a matter of false humility as French observed: 'it also has something to do with this deep-seated desire to hold on to as little responsibility as possible; after all, this time it paid off, but next time might be different'.

It is not just paediatric nurses who have to grapple with responsibility and accountability: parents and children are also inextricably linked in the responsibility barter game. Just as nurses are finding that they are responsible for ever increasing and invasive professional work, parents and children are also cajoled, and even encouraged, to take on ever more responsibility for their participation in health matters with healthcare workers (Alderson, 1993; Casey, 1993).

Responsibility of parents and children

Parents and children are asked to take on ever more responsibility without necessarily more obvious benefits or rights, except that it would appear that parents desire to continue with their parenting responsibilities and looking after their children, even in hospital (Casey, 1993). Parents see this not only as an ongoing burden but also as an ongoing parental right. Child healthcare, in this context, becomes a shared responsibility between various professional and non-professional adults.

The child, too, has a measure of responsibility. Traditionally children have been absolved from full responsibility on the premise that they are not capable of being fully responsible and, therefore, cannot be accountable for their acts. According to French (1993), in order to qualify as a player of the responsibility barter game the player must be a member of the moral community, which implies a particular level of moral and social development. Presumably, players once 'in the game' can be voted out, or temporarily disqualify themselves by virtue of disease, unconsciousness or lack of sobriety.

But children are changing and in some areas of their lives are completely competent and responsible and in other areas highly dependent on adult guidance. It is probably safest overall to consider children as lacking full moral and social competence, unless proven otherwise in a particular case. Children, additionally, have to prove that they possess relevant moral and social knowledge. In a practical example from health promotion, one could not hold children accountable for the maintenance of their own good dental health unless and until: first, they are capable of understanding the significance of daily oral hygiene and second, they have the requisite motor skills and intellectual ability to carry out daily dental hygiene and to plan an adequate nutritious diet.

One related question that troubles child sociologists, psychologists and moral philosophers concerns the nature of the loss of innocence (James & Prout, 1990; Archard, 1993). Rephrased, the argument suggests that we should be concerned that the price of being held responsible for our actions means an automatic loss of 'innocence'. Conversely, some would say that what a child does not know about harmful bacteria, for example, does not concern them; at least not directly. Personal knowledge brings with it personal responsibility and a loss of innocence.

French, however, points out that losing innocence is connected with gaining maturity and moral development, and that moral innocence is more akin to moral 'virginity' than moral purity. As he rightly points out, innocence is a matter of moral status, the status of someone not mature enough to be a fully 'paid-up' member of the moral community. It is not a condition that adults need, or indeed should yearn for, even though as he notes 'innocence . . . is only valued by those who no longer possess it' (French, 1993). Moreover, the world's children are only too aware of their losses and the altered state of childhood which they are forced to live out, often in grotesque circumstances. The children do not want the impossible nor are they hankering after an unrealistic dream. They want to attend school and to avoid serving in (adult) armies. They want to be free to play without the fear of mines and explosives, be free from adult prejudice and manipulation, and have equal access to healthcare (UNICEF, 2002). These are hardly the requests of unreasonable individuals.

Innocence absolves from responsibility, but only temporarily, as it is the duty and responsibility of adults who are collectively responsible before society, to instil in children the universal concepts of right and wrong and the nature of good and evil. Once 'moral innocence' is lost however, there is no going back: paradise can never be regained. Loss of moral 'virginity' is irrecoverable, since knowledge about oneself can only, by definition, be an active ongoing process (French, 1993). Thus, an asthmatic child taught by parents and the community paediatric nurse to use an inhaler, cannot go back on this knowledge and behave as if they never knew what to do in the event of an asthmatic attack.

Most children guard their autonomy and newly learnt skills, and do not see them as a loss of innocence so much as necessary growth and a move in the direction of maturity and self-determination. For this reason, many children who are taught how to use an inhaler, or to administer their own insulin, will not take kindly to giving up this responsibility to a teacher or camp director when the class goes on an outing or a camping trip. Additionally, with this responsibility comes the right to real – albeit limited – self-determination. It is difficult to argue with a child who has already been given responsibility as to why this responsibility should necessarily change and/or stop (Alderson, 1993).

Responsibility can therefore be seen as the most crucial element in the accountability equation, and one shared in proportion to moral development by children as well as adults. Thus, paediatric nurses in the course of their work are not only responsible for their own actions but also for the upholding of parents' ongoing responsibilities and the development of a child's own sense of responsibility. Accountability, for paediatric nurses, rests on a delicate balance of their professional responsibilities with those of parents and children, where the child's 'responsibilities' and self-determination will always be paramount, as it is the child who is at the centre of every paediatric nurse's concerns.

Conclusion

As the children of the world proclaim:

> Until others accept their responsibility to us, we will fight for our rights. We have the will, the knowledge, the sensitivity and the dedication. . . . We are the children of the world, and despite our different backgrounds, we share a common reality. We are united by our struggle to make the world a better place for all. You call us the future, but we are also the present.
> (UNICEF, 2002)

Paediatric nurses everywhere should heed this call by children for adults to play their full responsible role in society and to start promoting and protecting the rights of children everywhere. It is the children themselves who are setting the professional agenda and calling adults to account for their failings to protect them and guide them. The children are prepared to: 'promise to support the actions you [i.e. adults] take on behalf of children, [and] we also ask for your commitment and support in the actions we are taking, because children of the world are misunderstood' (UNICEF, 2002).

Chapter 10

Accountability and Clinical Governance in Learning Disability Nursing

Bob Gates, Mick Wolverson and Jane Wray

Introduction

In this chapter the issues of accountability and clinical governance and their relationship to the care of people with learning disabilities are explored. Throughout history, people with learning disabilities have been portrayed in various ways, e.g. being perceived as a menace to society, subhuman, an object of dread, burden or ridicule (Wolfensberger, 1972; Gates, 1997; Atherton, 2002). This negative portrayal has resulted in the inevitable vulnerability of this segment of society. Sadly, some people with learning disabilities continue to be misunderstood and subsequently experience prejudice and exclusion from their communities and society. In addition, it is well documented that this client group is susceptible to many forms of abuse, including physical, sexual, emotional and financial abuse (Moore, 2001). It is also known that this client group is, regrettably, more at risk of abuse from their carers (Moore, 2001) and that a strong philosophy of care and a sense of accountability are often absent from abusive environments (Sundram, 1986). This makes the issue of accountability and clinical governance for health and social care professionals who work with people with learning disabilities especially relevant.

A recent White Paper *Valuing People: A New Strategy for Learning Disability for the Twenty-first Century* (Department of Health, 2001c) has placed considerable emphasis on people with learning disabilities using mainstream services. The White Paper has clearly stated that people with learning disabilities have the same right of access to the range of healthcare services offered to the general population. In this respect, it acknowledges that services must respond to existing legislation to bring about the inclusion of people with learning disabilities. Therefore, in addition to guidelines surrounding nursing practice, legislation such as the Disability Discrimination Act 1995 and the Human Rights Act 1998 have placed enormous and far reaching obligations on professional practice and accountability. Legislation now exists that can, and undoubtedly will at some time in the future, be used against healthcare professionals or the organisations in which they work when people with learning disabilities face discrimination and prejudice.

Notwithstanding the implications of this legislation for all aspects of nursing practice, this chapter seeks primarily to address those issues specific to learning disability nurses. It is known that learning disability nurses work in many different settings and for different agencies. Their practice is often in disparate services spread over large geographical areas (Kent *et al.*, 2002). In addition, their roles are complex and range from care managers through to specialist clinical nurse practitioners (Alaszewski *et al.*, 2001). The difficulties posed by this complex interface of care and practice have prompted the United Kingdom Central Council for Nursing, Midwifery and Health Visiting (UKCC) (now replaced by the NMC) to issue specific guidance for learning disability nurses in the form of *Guidelines for Mental Health and Learning Disabilities Nursing* (UKCC, 1998a). This chapter now moves on to consider clinical governance, and how nurse practitioners are accountable for their practice through an ethical code of practice.

Clinical governance in learning disability nursing and guidelines for practice

A number of quality improvement and accountability procedures can be found currently within learning disability care settings. These include clinical audit, research, evidence-based practice, quality assurance, complaint procedures, risk assessment and management, clinical supervision, continuing professional development and lifelong learning (Figure 10.1).

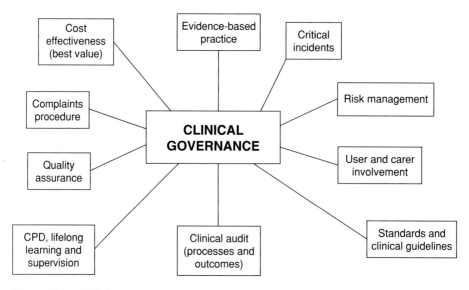

Figure 10.1 Clinical governance.

One interpretation of clinical governance is that it is a framework of pre-existing agenda that, when implemented, together ensure consistent excellence in care delivery. To some extent clinical governance is also concerned with changing elements of the culture of human services by challenging ingrained thinking and entrenched ways of working to improve standards of care. This is particularly relevant to some learning disability settings because of past evidence of long-standing problems in residential services caused by institutionalised ways of working. To paraphrase Mark Twain, by doing things the way you always did, you always get what you always got.

Clinical governance, therefore, is a change-process underpinned by a framework that draws together the various initiatives shown in Figure 10.1 and aims to assist practitioners in the maintenance and improvement of standards of care with the person with learning disabilities as the central focus. The framework of clinical governance and accountability is supported by professional self-regulation. Nurses are subject to standards set by their professional regulatory body, the Nursing and Midwifery Council (NMC). Professional self-regulation supports the process of clinical governance by requiring practitioners to monitor themselves and their own good practice. This is guided by three main principles:

- promoting good practice
- preventing poor practice
- intervening in unacceptable practice

It is thought that the application of the principles of clinical governance will 'provide an environment in which clinical excellence can flourish and high standards of patient care can be promoted' (UKCC, 2001a, p. 7).

Clinical governance requires all practitioners to regulate their practice, and fundamental to this concept is the development of appropriate standards and guidance for professional practice. These are encapsulated in a range of regulatory documents and codes produced by the UKCC. Documents such as the *Code of Professional Conduct* (UKCC, 1992a) *Guidelines for Professional Practice* (UKCC, 1996a) and *The Scope of Professional Practice* (UKCC, 1992b) have defined the responsibilities of registered nurses to patients, colleagues, employers, the public and themselves and are pertinent to all practising nurses, health visitors and midwives. At the time of writing this chapter only the *Code of Professional Conduct* has been updated by the NMC (2002b). However, the particular vulnerability of people with learning disabilities, and the documented history of abuse experienced by this client group (Moore, 2001), make it vital that each registered learning disability nurse safeguards and promotes the interests of people with learning disabilities. Next, this chapter briefly explores specific guidelines that have been constructed for mental health and learning disability nurses.

The document *Guidelines for Mental Health and Learning Disabilities Nursing – A Guide to Working with Vulnerable Clients* (UKCC, 1998a) explicitly recognises that specific guidance was needed for mental health and learning disability nurses because of the vulnerability of these client groups and because of the large number of practitioners working in the private or independent sector. The guidelines were designed to enhance awareness and understanding of accountability within an ethical, legal and professional context and cover pertinent issues such as:

- consent
- interdisciplinary working
- evidence-based practice
- advocacy
- autonomy
- relationships
- confidentiality
- risk assessment and management

Each of these is now briefly discussed.

Consent

In learning disability practice it is usually more helpful to talk of valid consent and this comprises three main elements:

- it is given by a competent person (or their representative)
- it is given voluntarily
- it is informed

Obtaining consent depends on the capacity and competence of the person with learning disabilities to understand the information given to them and to make an informed decision regarding their treatment or care. The capacity of people with learning disabilities to give consent may be hampered by a range of intellectual, physical, sensory or communication difficulties. These may significantly impair their ability to consent to treatment or care. Consequently, the best interests of the client and the duty of care must be assessed on an individual basis to ensure that any decisions made are reasonable, ethical and appropriate. Recently, the Department of Health has issued specific guidance entitled *Seeking Consent: Working with People with Learning Disabilities* (Department of Health, 2001d). It is advised that all students and practitioners familiarise themselves with this document and ensure that its requirements are assimilated into their practice.

Interdisciplinary working

'Providing care is an inter-professional and inter-agency activity and it should be based on co-operation, shared understanding and respect' (UKCC, 1998a, p. 10). Effective team working with clear lines of accountability is essential to ensure the health and well-being of people with learning disabilities. Client care and needs should always take priority over the resolution of interprofessional differences and conflicts. Interprofessional working is particularly important in view of the multi-agency context of care for people with learning disabilities. Increasingly, the lead agency in providing care will be social services and not health services (Department of Health, 2001c). Clearly there are significant challenges here for the practice of learning disability nursing and, whereas this speciality has a long history of interdisciplinary work, it will now have to face the challenge of inter-agency work.

Evidence-based practice (EBP)

EBP is a requirement that should be used to inform and develop all nursing practice in learning disability contexts. Nurses are responsible for continually updating their practice (as described in the *Code of Professional Conduct* (NMC, 2002)) and ensuring that the best possible evidence is taken into account when making clinical decisions. Muir Gray (1997) suggests that EBP 'is an approach to decision making in which the clinician uses the best evidence available, in consultation with the patient, to decide upon the option that suits the patient best' (p. 9). As with clinical governance, patient or client choices are central. EBP is also supported by the *Research Governance Implementation Plan* (Department of Health, 2001e) which aims to give guidance on good practice in health and social care and promote and enhance the research culture.

Advocacy

Clinical governance and accountability place safeguarding the interests of clients at the centre of practice and nursing care. However, within learning disability contexts it must not be assumed that the nurse necessarily knows what is best for the client as: 'advocacy is about promoting the clients' right to choose and empowering them to decide for themselves' (UKCC, 1998a, p. 14).

The literature on advocacy in learning disability remains divided as to whether advocacy is a legitimate and integral part of their nursing role (Cabell, 1992; Carpenter, 1992). Some authors have suggested that a conflict of interest militates against assuming such a role (Gates, 1994, 2001). The guidelines acknowledge this potential area of conflict and suggest that in most circumstances an independent advocate can provide more objective support to clients.

Autonomy

The guidelines for learning disability nurses support those of the *Code of Professional Conduct* (NMC, 2002b) and emphasise the importance of fostering client independence and autonomy. In practice, this means that decisions made by the multidisciplinary team should not only be in the client's best interests, but should also, where possible, involve the client. Central to the issues of promoting autonomy is the question of who holds the power to make decisions? *Valuing People* (Department of Health, 2001c, p. 26) has identified a governmental objective (no. 3) as being: 'To enable people with leaning disabilities to have as much choice and control as possible over their lives through advocacy and a person-centred approach to planning the services they need.'

Relationships

The guidelines again refer practitioners back to the *Code of Professional Conduct* (NMC, 2002b). This document states that: 'in the exercise of your professional accountability, [you] must avoid any abuse of your privileged relationship with patients and clients and of the privileged access allowed to their person, property, residence or workplace'.

All nurses are required to be aware of the power imbalance that exists between client and carer. Also, people with learning disabilities are particularly vulnerable to the misuse of power by their carers and registered nurses. In addition, *Practitioner-Client relationships and the prevention of abuse* (UKCC, 1999a) makes explicit the expectations of practitioners in therapeutic relationships and provides guidance on the prevention, detection and management of abuse that may occur.

Confidentiality

The UKCC *Guidelines for Professional Practice* (UKCC, 1996a) have provided advice on confidentiality and its importance within the therapeutic relationship. The *Guidelines for Mental Health and Learning Disabilities Nursing* (UKCC, 1998a) stated that a clear standard of confidentiality should always be explained to clients and documented, and that confidentiality should only be violated in exceptional circumstances with clear justification. These circumstances included when:

- the client consented
- it is required by law
- it is required by the order of a court
- it is in the public interest

The duty of confidentiality often poses specific problems for learning disability nurses when working with clients with a history of offending behaviour when they also and sometimes simultaneously have to liaise with colleagues in the criminal justice system.

Risk assessment and management

Risk management involves assessing the extent of risk relating to client care, care systems and the environment of care: 'The calculation of risk must be based on your knowledge, skills and competence and you are accountable for your actions and omissions' (UKCC, 1998a, p. 22). The guidelines acknowledge the difficulty in eliminating risk entirely and emphasise the nurse's responsibility for reducing risks to an agreed acceptable level. It is recommended that the reader refers to a recent publication on risk assessment and management that was based on empirical work conducted in the field of mental health and learning disability settings (Alaszewski *et al.*, 1997).

The document *Guidelines for Mental Health and Learning Disabilities Nursing – A Guide to Working with Vulnerable Clients* (UKCC, 1998a) has provided specific reference points for learning disability nurses, in addition to the existing guidelines and standards. Also, students and practitioners should be aware of professional misconduct and that there are a number of other documents providing guidance on nursing's accountable system, whereby practitioners can be removed from the register because they are a risk to the public. These include:

- *Protecting the public – an employers guide to the UKCC registration confirmation service for nurses, midwives and health visitors* (UKCC, 1999b)
- *Complaints about Professional Conduct* (UKCC, 1998b)
- *Reporting Misconduct – information for employers and managers* (UKCC, 1996b)
- *Reporting unfitness to practice – information for employers and managers. Issues arising from professional conduct complaints* (UKCC, 1996c)

The continuous maintenance and improvement of standards of knowledge and competence is essential to promote higher standards of care and to ensure that the practitioner is safe to practice in a constantly changing healthcare environment. Therefore, continuing professional development (CPD) seeks to ensure that the practitioner stays up to date and competent to practice. It encompasses informal private learning and reflection as well as formal courses and supportive mechanisms, such as mentorship, preceptorship and clinical supervision. It is suggested that CPD has the potential to make a significant contribution to clinical governance in that it recognises the importance of maintaining and improving clinical competence and knowledge. The UKCC's post-registration education and practice (PREP) framework is a CPD standard. In addition, clinical supervision (in *Supporting Nurses, Midwives and Health Visitors through Lifelong Learning*, UKCC, 2001b) contributes to risk assessment by providing opportunities for reflection on clinical practice (Wolverson, 2000).

The challenges of effectively implementing clinical governance in services for people with learning disabilities

Clinical governance comprises values and principles, such as effective leadership and communication, patient focus, commitment to quality, valuing all members of the healthcare team and continued professional development.

The pervasive challenge to implementing clinical governance in services for people with learning disabilities is engendering meaningful changes in the way services are delivered. Changing management and cultural mindsets can be seen to be an overarching challenge to implementing clinical governance. Many factors contribute to the difficulty of ensuring cultural change in learning disability settings, and these factors are listed in Box 10.1.

The potential barriers listed in Box 10.1 are generalised in that they are barriers hindering the implementation of clinical governance in all services and are applicable to all client groups. In relation to implementing clinical governance in services for people with learning disabilities, it is apparent that not only are all the barriers listed in Box 10.1 relevant, but that they are exacerbated by other factors that are more prevalent in learning disability services than perhaps in other services. These specific issues are outlined in Box 10.2 and each is to be discussed below.

Box 10.1   Potential barriers to the changes necessary for the implementation of clinical governance

- professional apathy
- short-term outlook of clinical governance
- poor awareness of clinical governance
- misinterpretation of the concept, e.g. a belief that clinical governance is merely a tool for management to monitor staff
- poor leadership
- a limited research portfolio on which clinical effectiveness should be based
- limited resources in terms of staff, time and support for those implementing clinical governance
- fragmented multidisciplinary working
- poor information systems
- poor communication
- change burnout – staff becoming overloaded by constant and incomplete change(s)
- theory – practice gap – when clinical governance remains a theoretical concept and fails to influence practice.
- scepticism – professionals doubt that clinical governance will achieve anything constructive
- maintaining motivation – initial enthusiasm for clinical governance can easily dissipate when seemingly insurmountable barriers exist
- priorities – clinical governance can be perceived to be peripheral when compared to more immediate concerns; also management and clinicians may lack agreement about priorities
- lack of consistency – different professionals such as doctors, nurses and researchers may have different interpretations and expectations of clinical governance
- the 'emperor's new clothes' – care staff may perceive clinical governance to be a transient fad and believe they have 'seen it all before'

Box 10.2   Specific significant barriers to implementing clinical governance in learning disability services

- fragmented partnership working
- difficulties in involving users and carers
- the diverse spectrum of needs associated with learning disability
- quality of life issues

Fragmented partnership working

Multi-agency partnership working has long been a laudable goal in the pursuit of providing quality care for people with learning disabilities. *Valuing people* (Department of Health, 2001c) has clearly identified strong partnership working as a priority, and has stated that there is great variability across the UK in terms of availability, consistency and quality of services. In addition, it is evident that services for people with learning disabilities are increasingly fragmented, with support being provided by a range of agencies such as social services, education and the agencies in the private, independent, not-for-profit and voluntary sectors. Weinstein (1998) has described this fragmentation as a consequence of a plethora of inter-linking issues that included conflict between agencies regarding values, unwillingness to accept responsibility, lack of shared aims or goals and lack of understanding of the roles and function of different professionals and agencies. Therefore, if clinical governance within learning disability nursing is to be effective then it will need to be implemented in creative and flexible ways to transcend the boundaries between agencies and professions.

User and carer involvement

A key component of the clinical governance framework is a commitment to include the views of service users and carers in the pursuit of quality care. This element of clinical governance is, in the case of people with learning disabilities, strengthened by the recent advent of person-centred planning (PCP) as outlined in *Valuing People* (Department of Health, 2001c). The benefits of user involvement are largely self evident and according to Lugon & Secker-Walker (2001) include:

- providing a mechanism for care staff to demonstrate accountability to the people they serve
- improved communication between users and staff
- a mechanism whereby the experience of users can influence decision making
- a facility for users to express their preferences
- a forum for expressing concerns
- a formal system for processing complaints

User involvement in clinical governance is vitally important because it can assist in making the process of care meaningful to people with learning disabilities, and offer ways of improving their lives. However, barriers to effective user involvement must be overcome. Notwithstanding this commitment, opportunities for meaningful consultation are rare, and the methods by which people with learning disabilities are involved in decision-making processes are often seen as 'tokenism' (Sang & O'Neill, 2001). Kelson (1997) has identified a number of other barriers that include:

- professional resistance (that is professionals may not value the contribution of users)
- concerns about confidentiality
- concerns regarding whether user and carer spokespeople are truly representative of the client group and the lack of support provided for people with learning disabilities to contribute to clinical governance programmes
- users and their representatives such as advocacy services, may also have agenda that are at odds with mainstream views

The spectrum of need

The term learning disability covers a spectrum of needs, from people with profound and complex healthcare needs, to people with a high functional ability who require limited support. It should be noted that the vast majority of people with learning disabilities are not ill, but that they may require social support at different times during their lives. Any system of clinical governance will need to be flexible enough to offer a significant quality of improvement for this diverse group of people.

Quality of life

A key component of the clinical governance framework, is quality improvement. The Royal College of Nurses (RCN, 1998a) has stated that: 'Quality improvement activities encompass standard settings and monitoring, clinical audit and evidence-based practice.'

This drive to continually improve the provision of services is obviously a commendable goal. However, the quality of life of people with learning disabilities can be extremely difficult to ascertain (Cummins, 1997). The improvement activities mentioned by the RCN (1998a), if applied to learning disability services, are often undertaken in subjective, bureaucratic and arbitrary ways that invariably achieve little meaningful improvement for service users. Ellis & Whittington (1993) have discussed how quality is notoriously difficult to define in the context of care delivery. Walshe *et al.* (2000) have stated that 'quality' can be used as an umbrella term to cover everything without changing anything in particular. Therefore, any clinical governance programme applied to people with learning disabilities needs to acknowledge the potential barriers to improving the quality of the service-user experience and provide solutions.

Solutions to the barriers associated with implementing clinical governance in learning disability services

The barriers identified above, that may prevent the implementation of clinical governance, will require a systematic and flexible approach to overcome them. The NHS clinical governance support team has recommended that services adopt a change model that incorporates four sequential stages as shown in Figure 10.2. This sequential process is known by the acronym RAID. It is proposed that the RAID model is a generalisable, systematic, flexible and problem-solving approach to implementing clinical governance. The NHS clinical governance support team has recommended that teams of staff apply the RAID model to their sphere of core activity as follows:

- Review
  A comprehensive fact-finding exercise should be undertaken, which should involve extensive consultation with all stakeholders in the service under review. This process should use qualitative methodology, e.g. in interviews with service users, carers and staff. The review should simply determine what is good practice in relation to current service and what is poor practice from the perspective of these key players. It should also ascertain what procedures and practices should be kept and what should be jettisoned.

- Agree
  Based on the findings of the review the clinical governance team should then agree on projects, which could improve the services offered to users. Examples of projects might include improving access to primary health-care, developing joint training packages between agencies, devising consensual agreed team goals and disseminating research to underpin evidence-based practice.

- Implement
  Projects identified will be implemented in care settings. It is expected that subgroups comprising users, carers, staff and key stakeholders will be responsible for the implementation of individual projects.

- Demonstrate
  The effectiveness of the identified clinical governance projects will be demonstrated through appropriate documentation. This will include follow-up user interviews and satisfaction questionnaires.

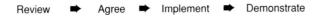

Review ➡ Agree ➡ Implement ➡ Demonstrate

Figure 10.2 Four sequential stages of change.

Table 10.1 Barriers and suggested solutions associated with the implementation of clinical governance in learning disability service settings.

Barriers	Leadership	Management	Cooperation	Inclusion	Mechanisms	Education
Apathy	Leaders as role models Transformational leadership Act as motivator	Personal development Reviews Explicit guidelines		Apathetic staff to be listened to	Portfolio development	Programmes to educate staff about the value of clinical governance
Short-termism	Identify processes to meet longer term goals	Provide direction and set short- and long-term goals	Involve staff in projects and working parties	Include staff in decision-making forums	Clearly define organisational goals	
Poor awareness of clinical governance	Inform staff regularly about clinical governance projects	Inform and monitor	Invite staff on to working parties		Develop robust communication network – newsletters and resource packs	Educate all staff and give regular updates
Misinterpretations	Reassure and inform	Reassure and inform Honesty and transparency		Expose staff to clinical governance agendas	Develop explicit information on clinical governance	Regular updates and information exchanges
Fashion	Demonstrate commitment	Issue long-term guidelines	Network with other services who can demonstrate the efficiency of clinical governance			
Poor leadership	Identify leaders for individual projects	Allow leaders to lead		Listen to staff and users		

Limited research base	Identify current research base and gaps	Allow staff to research pertinent areas	Conduct research in tandem with other agencies Encourage networking		Regularly disseminate latest research and journals	Raise awareness of research and induct staff into the process
Resources	Identify efficient working practices	Provide for the implementation of clinical governance by managing resources	Use external resources to access expertise			
Fragmented multi-disciplinary working	Draw terms together	Demarcate staff responsibilities	Encourage team building		Regular team meetings, consensually agreed modus operandi and goals	Joint training sessions
Poor information systems		Provide resources for information systems	Access the information systems of other agencies		Develop IT systems and sites	Team staff IT skills
Poor communication	Visible leadership, regular dissemination of information	Develop communication systems	Identify communications networks between agencies	Listen to the concerns of users and staff	Regular dissemination of written information	
Change burnout	Identify potential burnout victims and offer coping mechanisms	Set achievable short- and long-term goals		Listen to staff's concerns		

Table 10.1 (*cont'd*)

Barriers	Leadership	Management	Cooperation	Inclusion	Mechanisms	Education
Theory–practice gap	Act as role model and link between the two	Firmly place clinical governance in the care area	Access theoreticians and include them in the large area		Demonstrate via documentation examples of theory–practice link	
Scepticism	Act as role model Motivate and encourage Offer supervision	Regular personal development		Listen to the views of staff and provide solutions to their scepticism		Provide examples of the effectiveness of clinical governance
Maintaining motivation	Inspire and energise	Encourage and set goals		Include staff in project work		
Fragmented partnership working	Joint leadership	Joint management	Multi-agency working groups	Multi-agency representation in planning	Joint investment plans Shared budgets, partnerships, boards	Joint training days
User and carer involvement	Inspire and motivate	Representations in management teams	Utilise advocacy services	Listen to and respond to views	Representations on all decision-making groups	Joint training
Quality of life issues		Allow for democratic agreement on what constitutes quality of life		Demonstrate that the views of users are incorporated into service delivery	Development of meaningful evaluation documents	Educate staff about their role in enhancing the quality of life of users

The RAID approach offers an overarching model for implementing clinical governance. For clinical governance to flourish broad systems and specific mechanisms can be employed to overcome the barriers identified previously in Boxes 10.1 and 10.2. Table 10.1 outlines barriers and some proposed solutions associated with the implementation of clinical governance in learning disability service settings.

The causes of the barriers identified in Table 10.1 are multi-factorial and therefore any response to them will necessitate a multi-factorial response. The table demonstrates that clinical governance should permeate all elements of a service in order that coordinated responses can be developed. The identification of the challenges to implementing clinical governance demonstrates that instigating clinical governance is a complex and potentially difficult process. This daunting process can, however, be overcome by the use of the RAID approach and systematic, coordinated service responses. The benefits derived from implementing clinical governance are manifold and therefore the effort entailed in implementing this approach must be made. Clinical governance should not be implemented as a 'top-down' system as this can result in it remaining an abstract, theoretical concept that is resisted and rejected by staff. Clinical governance is a recognised mechanism for improving service provision. Nursing staff are accountable for their practice and therefore they should embrace clinical governance in their attempt to demonstrate accountability of their practice.

Conclusion

We have argued that the issues of accountability and clinical governance are particularly relevant to nurses who work with, and support people with learning disabilities and this is because of the potential for abuse, prejudice and discrimination. In learning disability contexts, clinical governance and the exercise of accountability have the potential to transform the care of people with learning disabilities in ways that can significantly impact on the quality of life for people with learning disabilities.

Chapter 11

Where does the Buck Stop?
Accountability in Midwifery

Rosemary Mander

Introduction

While being far from overexposed, the nature of accountability has been discussed regularly and authoritatively by nurses since the early 1980s. It is only relatively recently, though, that midwifery accountability has begun to attract the attention which it deserves. The reason for this belated attention may relate to midwives' long-standing concerns about their autonomy. This observation may not be as negative as it may first appear, as the association between accountability and autonomy, as I suggest below, is closer than may at first be apparent. This line of thought may, in fact, commend midwives. Their long-standing attention to autonomy suggests that, albeit indirectly, for all this time they may also have been contemplating their accountability. As Etuk (2001) establishes, the twin issues of autonomy and accountability are very much bound up with the midwife's professional identity.

In this chapter I probe where the midwife currently stands in relation to accountability. To do this, I draw partly on the nursing literature on accountability and compare it with the situation that has been identified as currently existing in midwifery. Some may rightly question the relevance of the nursing literature to the midwife, on the grounds that nursing and midwifery are fundamentally different occupational groups. By way of answer, I suggest that, first, nursing material is more relevant than other non-midwifery material. Second, the common nursing background, which at the time of writing still applies widely in the UK, enhances its relevance. In my discussion of accountability I will first of all seek to clarify the meaning of this term by briefly focusing on the various meanings which may be applied to it. Next, the vexed question of the one or ones to whom the midwife is accountable will be addressed. I will then examine the relationship between the two essential concepts already mentioned, accountability and autonomy. Having provided evidence for the assumption that midwives have yet to become fully accountable for their practice, I will consider what prerequisites are necessary to achieve that ideal state. Finally, I look beyond the achievement of full accountability to discuss its implications for the midwife.

What is meant by accountability?

This is one of those terms which may be interpreted in a wide variety of different ways. Accountability has come to mean almost all things to all people. This may be due to a general uncertainty about its precise meaning, beyond the obvious fact that it has something to do with counting. But there may be uncertainty about what it is that is being counted and who is doing the counting.

The confusion associated with this term is discussed by Greenfield (1975) as he attempts to 'gather the diverse strands encompassed by accountability into a more or less coherent form'. The result of his attempt is a focus on organisational accountability. This manifests itself as the extent to which North American healthcare facilities meet the needs of the various interest groups with whom they are associated. Immediately, the distinction between organisational and individual accountability becomes apparent. Unfortunately though, no sooner is this distinction clarified than it becomes clouded by the huge areas of overlap between the two concepts.

In this chapter, I concentrate mainly on the midwife's individual or personal accountability. The implications for the midwife of organisational and institutional accountability are inevitably mentioned when considering to whom the midwife is accountable and also the implications of accountability. The Nursing and Midwifery Council undervalues being accountable, defining it merely as: 'responsible for something or to someone' (NMC, 2002b, p. 10). This definition suggests that accountability 'to' and 'for' are alternatives. This is unlikely to be the case as a more useful dictionary definition of an accountable person indicates: 'someone who is accountable is completely responsible for what they do and must be able to give a satisfactory reason for it' (CDO, 2002). This definition emphasises the potential for disclosure or the preparedness to disclose the rationale for one's actions, which would bring us nearer to the meaning of this term.

The concept of preparedness to disclose implies a sense of being responsible or 'explicable' (Champion, 1991). The prerequisite concept of responsibility brings Champion to discuss the authority for action and then the need for that action to be within the individual's capabilities and area of expertise. Up to this point Champion has concentrated on the activity and the circumstances in which it is permitted. The other component of accountability, which she identifies, may be found in the possibility of needing to explain or justify that action. This applies in the sense of making the decision to undertake one course of action as opposed to another; the implication is that the consequences of both are known and understood. The need to explain or justify the choice which was made and the resulting actions may or may not arise, but accountability requires that the individual is always able to provide that explanation or justification.

Accountability, therefore, may be seen to be about decision making (Jones, 1994). The context within which these decisions are made is crucial to being accountable. For this the individual, working on the basis of his/her expert knowledge, must be able to exert his/her choice unfettered by trappings or constraints applied by others. The discussion by Champion is precisely applicable to the role of the midwife in the context of healthy childbearing. This is because it is midwives who are educated to care for women experiencing uncomplicated childbirth. In caring, they anticipate potential deviations from the physiological processes and initiate appropriate action in the case of any deviation. Champion's valuable consideration of accountability is not dissimilar to the meanings chosen by Greenfield. He defines the adjective 'accountable', from which accountability is derived, as: 'subject to giving an account; answerable or capable of being accounted for; explainable'.

Like Champion, Greenfield relates accountability and responsibility to the timing of the action. Responsibility is essentially anticipatory; it precedes the action in that it permits the midwife to assume authority for the care she is about to provide on the basis of her own expert knowledge and experience. The manner in which that responsibility is subsequently manifested is in the midwife's accountability. Greenfield maintains that that accountability incorporates her decision making at the time of the activity and the potential for justifying her decisions and actions on some later occasion.

This distinction in the timing of responsibility and accountability may appear to be little more than academic pedantry, until the implications are considered. Accountability cannot exist without responsibility having previously been granted, accepted and assumed. Whether that responsibility is accepted must depend on the individual in terms of their preparation through their education and experience. Thus, a midwife may not be held accountable, or have accountability imposed for an action, unless she was first given and had accepted, on the basis of her professional preparation, the responsibility for caring.

In his provocative examination of accountability Etzioni (1975) questions its reality. He argues, to begin with, that it may be used symbolically, as little more than a gesture. This serves to establish the moral credentials of the person making the gesture in terms of, for example, calling for healthcare providers' greater accountability to their clients. There is, according to Etzioni, no intention of implementing this form of accountability, but it may win over the client/group to the views of the one making the gesture.

In a similar vein, Etzioni continues by demonstrating the use of accountability as a ploy or pawn in the power politics of healthcare. He shows that the more powerful an occupational or professional group becomes, then the more others are accountable to them. This decidedly cynical approach to accountability may hold more than an element of truth. Its relevance to the context within which the midwife practises may yet become apparent.

To whom is the midwife accountable?

Having drawn on the work of Etzioni and Greenfield, which relates to organisational accountability, it is appropriate to begin my examination of who holds the midwife accountable. I begin by considering the institutional and legislative context within which he/she works.

Institutional accountability

Although not every midwife in the UK is employed within the National Health Service (NHS) or self-governing NHS trusts, a large majority are and some form of institutional accountability is required of them. It is possible that even the midwife who practises independently may be held accountable to those alongside whom he/she practises.

The role of midwives as employees inevitably requires them, through their contract of employment, to adhere to the policies of the organisation. Although they may perceive their role as being solely to provide care to the woman experiencing uncomplicated childbearing, their employers may require them to 'extend' their expertise in a particular direction.

An example of this phenomenon is illustrated in the writing of Hall (1999), who recounts and analyses two experiences of home birth. One of these was marred by the midwife's lack of confidence in the woman's ability to give birth healthily and happily without a room full of hospital technology. This midwife is likely to have been required by her employers to extend her practice in the direction of less technologically-based care. Even though it is fundamental to midwifery, this may not have been her area of choice.

In historical terms, the major organisational development which affected the midwife's accountability was the introduction of the NHS in 1948 (Tew, 1995). Prior to becoming employed by local authorities and hospital boards at this time, a large majority of midwives had been relatively independent practitioners, fully accountable to those whose births they attended. The advent of the NHS meant that more women were able and willing to give birth in hospital and that obstetricians began to become routinely involved in the care of healthy pregnant women. Thus, the orientation of midwives was changed. Their accountability came to be to their employers, who now paid their salary, and more and more to their obstetrical colleagues. Increasing obstetrical involvement soon lead to the 'as if' or 'just in case' routines and the 'cascade of intervention', which is associated with escalating medicalisation of the birth (Goer, 1995).

The need for more hospital facilities, including labour wards and postnatal beds, soon became apparent. Perhaps to justify the increasing number of maternity beds in the presence of a falling birth rate, a series of Government reports recommended increasing levels of hospital confinement. This scenario escalated and the numbers, status and power of obstetricians increased correspondingly and exponentially. So the scene was set for the 'technological revolution' which burst on to the obstetric stage in the early 1970s. This led to the observation that the midwife's accountability had been reduced, to the extent that she had been transformed into an 'obstetric nurse' (Walker, 1972, 1976).

The hierarchical organisational structures within which midwives continue to work serve only to diminish their accountability, as mentioned by Etzioni. A House of Commons Report (1992) and the Government's response to it (Department of Health, 1993c) do not appear to have fulfilled their promise to reverse this trend (Rothwell, 1996).

Accountability to the woman

Legislative accountability was originally intended to protect the public, and the legislative framework within which the midwife currently practises continues to have this aim. Although Jones (1994) attempts to distinguish them, accountability to the public and accountability to the client are synonymous. This is because, logically speaking, the public benefit must include, but is not equivalent to, the welfare of the individual woman for whom the midwife is caring. This may not be an easy concept to accept when the overall standard of that woman's care appears to be being determined by a book of *Midwives Rules* (UKCC, 2002) and a Supervisor of Midwives. It may be that accountability to the woman operates in two ways. The mode of operation discussed below, via the professional legislative framework, may be said to act indirectly, by the intervention of human and other agencies. A more direct form of accountability is that which midwives exercise in their day-to-day hands-on practice, involving the care of women, babies and families.

Personal accountability

It is cogently argued that in ethical terms the main form of accountability to carry any weight for midwives is their accountability to themselves. Jones (1994) indicates that this form of accountability is an unalterable fact of care. Caring according to one's own philosophy of life and acting consistently according to the demands set by one's own value system may call for a different standard of care than that required by any external agency. Tschudin regards this intensely personal sense of responsibility as comparable with the way 'religious people would say that they have to answer to God' (1989). Smith (1981) supports the crucial and fundamental nature of personal accountability, because it operates at all times, throughout the life of any healthcare provider, unlike the few occasions on which the midwife may be asked to give account of her actions to an outside body. I would argue that this personal form of accountability is the highest form, underpinning all other forms of accountability, in that being accountable to oneself is an essential prerequisite to being able to be accountable to any other person or agent.

While contemplating the significance of personal accountability we should consider the effects of the dichotomy between personal accountability and external accountability on learning. In the event of a mistake by a care provider personal accountability might, through reflection, facilitate learning, personal growth and greater maturity. On the other hand external accountability, through a legislative framework, may lead to little more than disciplinary action.

Professional accountability

Tschudin (1989), in discussing the various forms which nursing accountability may take, describes the legislative framework through which the nurse's accountability to the public operates. In the opening years of the twentieth century the equivalent midwifery framework reached the statute book two decades earlier than that for nurses, against a background of jingoistic public concern at the lack of suitable manpower to fight popular colonial wars. Midwives were considered essential to solve the problems of infant mortality and morbidity, in order to lay the foundations for a healthy population from which recruits could be drawn (Robinson, 1990), but the public still needed protection from unsafe and incompetent practitioners. Legislation was sought which would provide adequate protection.

This legislation eventually emerged for England and Wales in the form of the first Midwives Act (1902). In spite of its well-known flaws (Donnison, 1988), this legislation recognised the special position of the midwife compared with other carers, in terms of her accountability for her actions. Since the beginning of the twentieth century the solitary nature of the midwife's practice and her role in prescribing and administering certain medicines have been regarded as putting the midwife in need of a specific regulatory framework.

This framework is in the form of the statutory *Midwives Rules* and the non-statutory but otherwise equivalent *Code of Practice* (UKCC, 2002). Such a framework causes one to question the extent to which the midwife is truly accountable, as these rules relate to clinical care decision making, among other areas. Newson (1986), having established the original need for the *Midwives Rules* as relating to training needs and the protection of families from unsafe practitioners, recognises the questions they raise about the midwife's accountability. She further asks whether these rules continue to be necessary. In answer to her question, she indicates the variation in midwives' competence 'from excellent to less than satisfactory'. The continuing practice of 'less than satisfactory' midwives is a sad reflection on midwifery supervision and our systems of basic and continuing midwifery education. It is hardly a justification, though, for what may be perceived to be a legislative straitjacket. Although midwives such as Newson clearly regard the rules as a supportive framework within which the midwife may practise safely, it may be that the existence of this framework constitutes more of a threat to midwifery, by limiting accountability, than a support to safe practice.

Closely linked with the *Rules and Code of Practice* is the role of the Supervisor of Midwives, described by Duerden (2002):

When practice problems are identified, Supervisors of Midwives provide support and guidance to midwives creating an opportunity to develop practice. This is through the facilitation of a period of supervised practice during which the Supervisor of Midwives ensures that the midwife has the necessary knowledge and skills.

The potential and real difficulties in the relationship between the midwife and the Supervisor of Midwives are well known (Hunter, 1998; Beech & Thomas, 1999).

Isherwood (1988, 1989) maintains that in a supportive situation this relationship may be 'close and cooperative'. It is easy to understand, however, that it may deteriorate into being 'confrontational' when the midwife is called to account to her supervisor for the standard of her practice. Isherwood relates that, in such destructive relationships, it is not only the midwife who suffers, but also the client, through the more restricted service which she may be offered. The questionnaire survey by Burden & Jones suggests that the midwife's perception of the judgemental nature of midwifery supervision is gradually beginning to change (2001).

It may be that midwifery supervision is the more acceptable face of the midwife's professional accountability. The other side, that is the disciplinary procedures, is detailed by Symon (2002). Serious complaints by clients, police and employers are screened and dealt with by the NMC, to assess whether the charges against the midwife are proven. If so, the Professional Conduct Committee must decide whether they should be cautioned or their name be removed from the professional register on a temporary or a permanent basis.

There is one question which inevitably arises out of this examination of the midwife's accountability. This is whether, for traditionally autonomous practitioners such as midwives, the very existence of these statutory bodies and the associated legislative framework serves by to reduce the need for them to regard themselves as accountable?

Hierarchy of accountability

It may be argued that personal accountability, through which one has to justify one's actions to oneself, is the highest order of accountability. This may be because of the continuing nature of personal accountability or perhaps because of the tendency for the demands we make of ourselves to be higher than those other people make of us. Does accountability in such circumstances equate with our conscience? The lower order forms of accountability, such as the organisational form, may have more easily apparent consequences in terms of the potential for disciplinary action and implications for employment. For this reason they may be more readily discussed and reported. It is being suggested here that they certainly pale into relative insignificance compared to personal accountability.

Accountability and autonomy

I have already attempted to define accountability and its significance in midwifery. Its relationship to autonomy is close and complex; to attempt to disentangle them is no mean feat. It may be that these concepts constitute two sides of the same coin, making them effectively inseparable, but still deserving separate scrutiny due to their differing contribution to informing the midwife's role (Mander, 1993). I hope to disentangle the relationship between these concepts in this section.

In discussing accountability up to this point, it has appeared to be a controlling or limiting phenomenon, to the extent that it may constrain the actions of the midwife. Even the possibility of having to explain or justify one's actions carries a strong implication that there is at least the potential for an error to have been made. Thus, accountability appears to be a somewhat more negative concept. This impression of the relative negativity of accountability is reinforced by our first glance at the definition of autonomy as: 'self-government or the right of self-government; self-determination' (OED, 2002). This definition carries with it the implication that autonomy is a permissive, liberating phenomenon. It may be regarded as being as positive as accountability is negative; as Vaughan (1989) observes: 'Some people have interpreted autonomy as meaning total freedom to act.' This clearly cannot apply if chaos is not to ensue.

Some of the limitations on autonomy may be apparent within the dictionary definition. When rights to 'self-determination' are conferred or assumed it is necessary to question 'by whom?' The right to self-determination cannot exist in a vacuum, as it carries implications for those who award it, as well as for others; some negotiation may be necessary before a 'right' is generally agreed. Vaughan and Champion point out other limitations on the 'total freedom' hypothesis. These limitations may be categorised according to their internality or externality to the would-be autonomous individual. The former, or 'personal' autonomy, focuses on the way in which autonomy only exists within the boundaries of competence, which in turn are created by the individual's finite knowledge base. The more external form, or 'structural' autonomy, implies the hierarchical or bureaucratic organisation within which most midwives practise and which inevitably limits and constrains their freedom of decision making.

In an attempt to move forward this simplistic categorisation of autonomy, Vaughan pleads for 'attitudinal autonomy' which relates to the individual's perception of themselves as an autonomous and accountable practitioner. Attitudinal autonomy may be construed as having the self confidence to take appropriate decisions and to be prepared to accept any consequences which may ensue.

A significant contribution to the literature on accountability in midwifery is found in the classic work of Walker (1972, 1976). The major focus of this research project was the role of midwives, but it illuminated their autonomy in midwife-obstetrician relationships as well as their accountability. Walker shows how the distinction in roles had become blurred in the minds of some of those involved. This blurring had given rise to conflicts between the expectations and the practice of care. Whereas each midwife saw themselves as accountable for the care of women experiencing uncomplicated childbirth, it was the medical staff who saw themselves as having overall responsibility and being able to exercise it at will. Walker's work showed that midwives understood the extent to which they were accountable, but that their medical colleagues were less clear about midwives and their role. It may be questioned whether the research which Walker undertook in the early 1970s has any continuing significance. That it does is supported by more recent, though less precisely relevant, studies by Robinson *et al.* (1983), Kitzinger *et al.* (1990) and Brownlee *et al.* (1996).

The autonomy of those involved in the childbearing experience was clearly established in the Health Committee Report (House of Commons, 1992) and the Government response (Department of Health, 1993c). Although these documents preferred the words 'choice' and 'control', they provide answers to the vexed question of the needs and wishes of both the woman and the midwife with regard to autonomy. These reports established the autonomy of the woman to the extent that she is to be the central decision-maker in matters relating to her care. The other major principle on which this report is founded is the accountability of the midwife, to the extent that maternity care will be midwife-led. The provision for the midwife to consult with obstetricians concerning the relatively small number of women in whom problems are identified was intended to continue to feature. Although these reports proved to be far from 'self-executive', their existence has fuelled unprecedented changes in the midwife's perception of her role and practice.

The relationship between autonomy and accountability may be summarised in terms of two concurrent personal monitoring systems. Using the analogy of a continuum of internality/externality, autonomy is the more internal while accountability is, perhaps only marginally, the more externally oriented. The relationship between autonomy and personal accountability may be so close on this continuum as to be barely perceptible.

What are the prerequisites for accountable midwifery practice?

I have already referred to the significance of the individual midwife's knowledge-base in achieving accountability. Because accountability is about decision making, the knowledge from which those decisions are derived is of fundamental importance. The need for midwives to avoid the danger of becoming complacent in their knowledge-base is similar to the need, emphasised by Champion, for nurses to 'develop and maintain their knowledge'. The development and nature of the midwifery knowledge-base may also merit attention. For too long this has been founded on superiors' whims and medical information (Mander, 1992a).

A supposed panacea which has been introduced to the UK healthcare system to address some of its multiplicity of problems is the oddly named clinical governance. This concept draws on two forms of research in order to provide a sound knowledge-base to achieve its aims (Sargent, 2002). These are clinical audit and evidence-based practice. As Sargent shows, this reductionist approach to care serves to downgrade practice, effectively, to 'midwifery by numbers'. The human 'knowledges' on which midwifery has traditionally drawn, such as intuition, occupational experience, personal knowledge and gut feeling, may no longer be permitted to feature in the repertoire of the accountable practitioner.

What are the implications of the midwife being accountable?

Although I have not presented accountability as the answer to all of midwifery's problems, I have not yet considered the serious disadvantages which some may prefer not to contemplate. A problem which would arise were midwives to assume full accountability is that their employers would cease to accept vicarious liability, as at present, through the master/servant relationship between employer and employee. A midwife being fully accountable would involve her being answerable to her clients for the decisions taken prior to providing care. The spectre of litigation assumes a more solid form when a midwife considers that he/she, like his/her medical colleagues, may be held personally responsible for any perceived or actual error of care. Without a willingness to accept this ultimate responsibility, midwives could not regard themselves as fully accountable. Having raised the spectre of litigation, the midwife's responsibilities in improving the present complaints system become apparent. Were this system to become less confrontational, as suggested in the Health Committee Report (1992), this grotesque phenomenon would assume more manageable proportions.

It is necessary to emphasise that there may be a price to pay for accountability. This price is the cost of taking risks, personally, professionally and organisationally, and accepting the consequences of our own actions. Risk-taking is an essential component of learning and the personal growth which ensues. For this reason accountability is as essential for midwifery to mature into a genuine profession as it is for each individual midwife to become genuinely professional.

Conclusion

Drawing on both midwifery and nursing literature, I have outlined the position of the midwife in relation to accountability. The multiplicity of agencies to whom midwives may be held accountable suggests that their accountability is severely curtailed by the legislative framework within which they practise. Research which focuses more on midwives' declining autonomy, has shown that their accountability is similarly threatened. Midwives through their organisation of midwifery education and midwifery research have it within their power to correct this serious deficit in their professional role. Before seeking to assume complete accountability every midwife must be comfortable with the increased personal costs which this would require them to bear.

In summary, it is clear that midwives are moving forward in the direction of greater accountability. In this journey they have both help and hindrances, some of which require action by midwives themselves.

While this chapter uses 'she' or 'her' to indicate 'the midwife', this is for descriptive ease only and the authors and editors of this book recognise the contribution of both male and female nurses to the profession.

Chapter 12
Accountability in Community Nursing

Sarah Baggaley with Alison Bryans

Introduction

A wide range of meanings has been attributed to the concept of community. Core ideas generally have a positive tone, and include notions of interdependence or connectedness and belonging, rather than mere proximity or simply sharing physical space.

What, therefore, is the relevance of these meanings to nurses working in the community? First, it is necessary for community nurses who wish to be successful in their practice to seek to understand and embrace the character of a community in which they work, and the significance of this for its inhabitants. This involves awareness of the total environment, a working knowledge of a social model of health (Williams *et al.*, 1993), and a flexible and holistic approach to healthcare, rather than too narrow a focus. Second, the working environment is filled with a vast array of other workers – nurses and others with whom community nurses must cooperate in order to achieve the best deal for their clients. Special skills in networking (which include identification and use of available resources), are essential, as well as good interpersonal skills. Third, as well as being accountable to individual clients, to line management and to the Nursing and Midwifery Council (NMC) the community nurse may be said to have a particular responsibility towards the community itself.

As issues of accountability for community nurses clearly cross the national boundaries reference will be made throughout this chapter to policy publications from all parts of the United Kingdom. However, the detailing of the differences in approach from the different countries is not within the scope of this account.

Organisational and policy issues affecting the accountability of community nursing

Recent and continuing change is the background and the ensuing challenge for the profession, requiring nurses to review and to maintain accountability for their practice. Therefore, organisational and policy issues within primary healthcare, which have certain implications for accountability in nursing practice, will be discussed briefly.

Throughout the 1990s the approach to healthcare policy was to enhance primary care, with the pace of change gathering momentum into the new millennium. Although the change of priority was welcomed by many community nurses, the reforms in the early part of the decade left some concerns as to the direction care in the community was taking, with the emphasis on seeking to change people's health behaviours primarily through screening and professional advice. Concerns were expressed at the potential demise of primary prevention in favour of secondary screening, evidenced by the General Practice (GP) contract (Department of Health, 1990); with a GP-centric service at odds with World Health Organisation (WHO) directives, where nurses are seen as crucial to action strategies (Williams *et al.*, 1993; WHO, 1986).

The advent of a Labour Government in 1997, however, changed the ethos in favour of community nursing, as the longer-term benefits of their skilled work plus their role in public health was acknowledged through a series of publications (Acheson, 1998; Department of Health, 1997; Home Office, 1998; Department of Health, 1999d; NHS Executive, 1999a; Scottish Executive Health Department, 2001b). Now there is a real climate of opportunity for community nurses to play a full and leading role in the delivery of care, as they are key to much of the agenda. Change also brings a challenge to traditional boundaries and working practices for all staff, with a demand to develop more flexible ways of working that make best use of the skills and knowledge of all team members (Sines, 2001). Increasingly, there are developments in nursing teams incorporating not only skill mix, but also integrated teams of nurses from the different disciplines aiming to share their expertise to provide effective care for clients by utilising individuals' specialist skills, facilitating shared objectives in health promotion and avoiding overlap of resources (Appleby & Sayer, 2001).

Since devolution and the establishment of a Scottish Parliament in 1999 Scotland has increasingly taken a distinctive approach to health, both in terms of organisation and in the priorities for health. Although the plan for the NHS in Scotland, laid out in *Designed to Care* (Scottish Executive Health Department, 1998), shares common goals with the rest of the UK, the organisational structures, particularly in the community, are substantially different, with the development of primary care trusts from April 1999 and the establishment of local healthcare cooperatives (LHCC) based on general practices (Hopton & Heaney, 1999). The focus for improving health in Scotland has been more clearly and quickly articulated through the public health agenda (Clarke *et al.*, 2001). In many ways the approach in Scotland is more radical, particularly in the field of public health and primary care, with the appreciation that Scotland's health compared to that of other European nations is poor and the life expectancy shorter. The heartening promise is that 'we are committed to making the NHS a national health service, not a national illness service' (Scottish Executive Health Department, 2000a, p. 13).

This emphasis on public health has been a tonic for health visitors in particular, who now feel that at last their worth has been recognised, but the onus is on them to deliver. The development of a public health approach to care, with partnerships with individuals, families and communities at its heart requires a clear accountable framework for practice. This is an area that will be returned to later in the chapter.

Current issues in community nursing

Resource allocation and skill mix

A systematic approach, with staffing levels among community nurses being based on health needs, rather than on the continuation of historical provision, is imperative to increase accountability of the profession through justifying its practice, both to the public it serves and to its employers who purchase its skills.

An example of this was the proposal from the NHS Management Executive (1993) that £40m a year could be saved by halving the numbers of G-grade district nurses and replacing them with less qualified or untrained staff. The swift reaction from the profession highlighted their understanding not only that it was a direct attack on jobs but also that it would undermine the Government's attempt to expand and improve community services. Cowley (1993) demonstrated that the review was based on flawed beliefs regarding the simplicity of nursing practice. It ignored the need for professional judgement, the variety of skills and the level of decision making in continuing assessment and practice.

This perception has been endorsed by McIntosh *et al.*'s (1999, p. 89) exploration through research into district nursing skills, which suggested that: 'the nature and range of skills in use in district nursing have been seriously underestimated. As a consequence changes in grade mix have been made on a set of assumptions rather than on evidence.'

McIntosh *et al.* question whether senior management is in a position to make satisfactory judgements on the mix of grades required, and suggest that it is only at the level of the nursing team that decisions on grade mix can be made, following careful assessment of patient need by the team leader, who appraises the appropriateness of skills and knowledge of all team members.

Delegation in skill mix

Delegation is integral to working in current nursing teams, and the early findings from McIntosh's timely study showed that the considerable insight and skills of senior staff were built up over time, leading to an understanding of junior staff's capabilities and skill levels. Senior staff at G or H grades demonstrated wider assessment skills, in particular identifying potential risk factors, skills not noted at more junior levels. From this broad assessment they were able to delegate the care of patients in a responsible and appropriate manner (McIntosh *et al.*, 1999).

The Community Practitioners and Health Visitors Association's professional briefing concerned with delegation and professional accountability (Forester, 2002) utilises Bergman's (1981) model to identify levels of accountability and its component elements of ability, responsibility and authority. Accountability for any work undertaken remains with the individual who had the authority to delegate it to another member of the team. The responsibility for ensuring the work is done lies with the person who agrees to accept the task, and that person is accountable for accepting that they have the competence required to undertake the role. This emphasises that delegation is a two-way process. The Nursing and Midwifery Council (2002b) *Code of Professional Conduct* provides guidance on delegation in a team in clauses 4.5, 4.6 and 6.2, stating:

> When working as a member of a team, you remain accountable for your professional conduct, any care you provide and any omission on your part. You may be expected to delegate care delivery to others who are not registered nurses or midwives. You remain accountable for the appropriateness of the delegation, for ensuring that adequate supervision or support is provided. To practice competently, you must possess the knowledge, skills and abilities required for lawful, safe and effective practice without direct supervision. You must acknowledge the limits of your professional competence and only undertake practice and accept responsibilities for those activities in which you are competent.

This articulates the accountability mandated by the professional body and thus expected by society. The profession formally registers practitioners through the NMC and advises its practitioners on standards of professional conduct through a variety of publications. It is the duty of every nurse to be totally conversant with the standards of care and scope of professional practice laid down by the NMC.

The above extract from the *Code of Professional Conduct* also makes explicit that nurses can be held accountable not only for activities but also omissions. Cowley & Andrews (2001) use scenarios to illustrate where accountability lies in the case of failure to detect problems within health visiting caseloads, when clients may not have been seen by practitioners over a lengthy period of time. In their discussion they highlight the need to establish what is an acceptable standard of practice for health visitors who have responsibility for an assigned population.

Botes notes that health visitors are: 'employed to be accountable for identifying vulnerable families within a universal service and providing them with the help they need' (Botes, 1998, p. 221). She continues, saying that the accompanying process is also identifying those families who have available resources and so may be left to ask for professional support when they need it. This would mean that the health visitor would not seek to make contact with these families, believing that the families themselves would contact the health visitor if they had any concerns. It takes a highly skilled practitioner to be able to make this assessment on the needs of all families on their case load and get it right.

Apart from the need for clear professional judgement, Cowley & Andrews also state that it is not only the individual practitioner or service commissioner who is responsible for determining an acceptable standard, but also what is determined to be a reasonable standard of practice by the profession. They continue, saying:

> There is a need for a credible body of professional opinion against which the actions of individual practitioners or service plans made by trusts can be judged. The source of such a body of professional opinion is, at present, also unclear.   (Cowley & Andrews, 2001, p. 141)

This clearly falls within the remit of the clinical governance agenda (see below).

Legal and professional issues in community nursing

Nurses have been attracted to working in the community for a variety of reasons, but high on the list is the feeling that they have greater autonomy and professional responsibility, allowing for more freedom in their decision making and determining the care that they provide. Independent professional practice, valued by community nurses, brings with it a greater responsibility to maintain the highest standards of professional competence. The risk of failure to deliver optimum care can be higher when individuals have a greater degree of autonomy, especially as so much of care in the community is unobserved activity.

A welcome development is clinical supervision, endorsed and encouraged both at Government level and by the profession (Department of Health, 1999c; Kohner, 1994). A flexible approach to clinical supervision is suggested by Dickerson, who sees it as 'a means to promote and develop quality patient care and confident accountability' (Dickerson, 1997, p. 190). Walsh (2001) cites a wealth of evidence indicating positive benefits for nurses in terms of professional development and ensuring quality of care, both of which are integral to an individual practitioner's accountable practice. The need to engage in effective clinical supervision is one of the professional challenges for community nurses, requiring an investment of skill and time. Sines (2001) argues that it should encompass positive and supportive feedback. Clinical supervision should not, however, be seen as a managerial tool for performance review.

As clinical supervision is not mandatory, practice nurses who are directly employed by GPs may face further challenges in finding regular time for reflection on their practice in this manner. Some may have difficulty in justifying time away from patient contact. However, since the integration of general practices into larger primary care organisations such as the LHCCs in Scotland, practice nurses may have an increasing sense of belonging to wider nursing communities, and greater opportunities to access support and ideas (Saunders, 2001).

Clinical governance

The need for evidence to inform understanding of complex nursing skills and assessment has never been greater. The ability to articulate the complexities of practice clearly, and identify the evidence of its effects is at the core of accountability. Historically, health visitors, in particular, have suffered from lack of understanding from other professionals about what they do; so making their skills and judgement visible and explicit was seen as a way of enhancing professional standing and convincing people of their worth. Today it is even more imperative for reasons of accountability at a time of great change in the nature and delivery of care. Health visitors may not feel appropriately valued, but as Kendall so succinctly states:

> there is an obvious managerial response: if you think that your service is a valuable one that should be retained, prove it – and prove it in cost terms, in clinical effectiveness terms and preferably in public health terms as well.
> (Kendall, 1999, p. 35)

Unless the case can be made the quality of service and the protection of the public may be diminished. Over their time in office the Labour Government has emphasised the importance of quality in the health service and nurses will play a key role in this process (Department of Health, 1997; Department of Health, 1998; Scottish Executive, 1998). The concept of clinical governance is at the core of this drive for quality, and accountability is at the heart of clinical governance. The Department of Health defines clinical governance as:

> a framework through which NHS organisations are accountable for continuously improving the quality of their services and safeguarding high standards of care by creating an environment in which excellence in clinical care will flourish.
> (Department of Health, 1998, p. 33)

Allen (2000) sees three strands to clinical governance in primary care: increasing the accountability of the professionals involved to local communities, to the NHS hierarchy and to other team members. The variety of activities entailed in clinical governance includes: clinical audit, research and development, risk management, quality initiatives, clinical effectiveness activities, team working and improved communication (Clarridge *et al.*, 2001; Adams & Forester, 2002).

There remains the tension of trying to satisfy equally the issues of accountability for each of the three strands as identified by Allen, that of local communities, management and other team members and also the profession, since there can be conflicts of interest between these groups. Allen sees the need to prioritise some aspects and feels accountability to team members is the 'bedrock' of clinical effectiveness in primary care, so good team working with leadership that can address the various agenda for change is essential (Adams & Forester, 2002). Allen thinks that the NHS hierarchy will be satisfied through attention being given to a mixture of centrally established clinical issues and locally identified issues in the health improvement plans, so attention to accountability to local communities may be reduced in the short term.

Although there is some lay representation at various levels of primary care organisation, the NHS faces challenges in trying to involve users in service planning. Community nurses work very much at the interface between the public and lay carers, on one hand, and management and other professionals on the other, and this creates particular dilemmas with regard to accountability. Health visitors, in particular, have striven for many years to clarify their remit as a profession that seeks to bridge the gap between professionals and recipients of care, consistently claiming an advocacy role and aiming to use health visiting expertise to represent and empower clients; not a straightforward task. The developing public health agenda, and the inclusion of health visitors and other community nurses on primary care management groups such as local health community councils, may afford opportunities to channel communication more effectively to local decision makers. This may ensure that the professions' perception of the causes of health problems, gained through their local knowledge, and their accessibility and acceptability to local communities, will be understood and considered in the planning of service provision.

Clinical effectiveness and evidence-based practice

Clinical effectiveness entails nurses (and others) utilising the best available evidence in their practice, the outcome of which is then evaluated, as part of an audit process. An integral aspect of the commitment to lifelong learning is another part of clinical governance. This involves not just attending study days; it is more a way of continually reflecting on practice and seeking ways to find examples of initiatives that have been effective for others. Therefore, ways of disseminating and sharing the knowledge of achieved effectiveness is also part of clinical effectiveness. What is equally apparent is that the evidence has to be used in a sophisticated manner so that the context of care is incorporated into the decision-making process (Closs & Cheater, 1999).

Consultation with the client and carers is essential to reach a decision that is the most suitable for the client's needs (Clarridge *et al.*, 2001). Kendall (1999) addresses the specific evidence base for health visitors' work with a well argued assessment of utilisation of research. She notes that there is still some way to go before the authorities are convinced of the worth of paradigms of research that reflect the qualitative characteristics of health visiting, and gives the examples of reassurance to an exhausted first time mother and confidence building in a group of single teenage parents.

Many authors (Bergman, 1981; McClymont *et al.*, 1986; Glover, 1999) indicate that responsibility can only be a reality if the professional has the authority to act. Clearly the authority is invested in community nurses for much of their practice through education and knowledge but as McClymont *et al.* (1986, p. 88) point out: 'responsibility without authority undermines professional autonomy and creates frustration'. There can be problems if a community nurse assesses that an individual needs a variety of services but the authority to provide them is outside their jurisdiction. It is perhaps surprising then that the *Code of Professional Conduct* only defines accountability as 'responsible for something or to someone' (NMC, 2002b, p. 10).

Health visitors, Kendall states, are often in a position of responsibility without the authority. Kendall argues that this may mean that research cannot be put into practice to improve health. She argues further that health visitors must be empowered to discover the best possible evidence for practice and that this implies investment by management in training in critical thinking, evaluating research, and other research skills, as well as being given time away from clinical work (Kendall, 1999). It is an argument that would apply to all community nurses.

In relation to the practice nurse, Saunders (2001) states that access to information technology must be available, along with the skills to locate and identify evidence-based material in the many databases currently available. Currently the Community Practitioners and Health Visitors Association (CPHVA) is pursuing a high profile campaign to 'make IT happen' following a survey of members to find out what access they have to the internet and email. The aim of the campaign is that every community nurse will have desktop access to a computer and access to the internet and NHS directory services. They highlight that provision is still patchy and that some NHS employers remain slow in empowering staff to benefit from the health information revolution (CPHVA, 2001).

Role developments

The roles of nurses in the community have been expanding dramatically throughout the recent period of change. Buttigieg (1997) argued that it was increasingly apparent that a primary care led NHS would only become a reality if nursing roles were enhanced, and the evidence today demonstrates that this is happening. Concern about cost effectiveness, demand for enhanced roles by nurses, an increased GP workload plus greater expectations from patients themselves, alongside changing healthcare legislation, have brought about these changes (Chapple *et al.*, 2000; Shaum *et al.*, 2000; Pritchard & Kendrick, 2001).

Nurses have taken advantage of current circumstances and as well as significantly expanding their role in general practice through nurse led services, they have been part of, and in some areas have led services within the Personal Medical Services (PMS) Primary Care Act pilot schemes (Gardner, 1998; Chapple *et al.*, 2000). Following the NHS (Primary Care) Act 1997 these schemes have emerged, particularly in deprived inner city areas, where they offer alternative services to vulnerable groups in accordance with the Government's aim to reduce health inequalities and tackle social exclusion (Walsh, 2001). Other forthcoming policy directives include walk-in centres and healthy-living centres, which also offer potential for role expansion.

At the time of writing, the new general medical services (GMS) contract is under negotiation. The Department of Health envisages:

> whilst it is too early to anticipate the exact contents of the new contract it is clear that there will be a considerable impact on nursing. Whatever the new contract brings there is a clear certainty that community nurses will have to develop both their core and specialist skills, and integrate with a wide range of multidisciplinary teams. The emphasis is on increasing flexibility of working with 'greater freedom to innovate and make decisions about services and the care that they provide. This will need to be matched with accountability for individual professional judgement and the use of best available evidence'.   (Department of Health, 2002b, pp. 7, 10)

This key message equates with Gardner's statement that accountability is one of the key areas that requires attention by community nurses if they are to take up the challenge of the opportunities on offer. Gardner, who has had experience of leading a primary healthcare team, feels that accountablity is: 'one of the major weaknesses of our profession. Historically it has been too easy to blame someone else, whether that is the trust, the nurse manager, the practice manager or the GP' (Gardner, 1998, p. 22). In the years since Gardner delivered that message, however, it is possible to see, through keeping up to date with journals such as *Community Practitioner*, where examples of innovative practice and leadership demonstrate the changing roles and adaptability of community nurses, indications that some are developing creative practice.

In line with accountable practice, it is important to take account of patients' views, and research indicates patient satisfaction with nurse led services as well as demonstrating that nurses can effectively manage a minor illness service in general practice (Chapple *et al.*, 2000; Shaum *et al.*, 2000; Pritchard & Kendrick, 2001). As the authors conclude, development of these specific services may readily be replicated elsewhere, although there are many other examples of changing roles. The creation of NHS Direct in England and Wales in 2000 and NHS 24 in Scotland in 2002 (24-hour help lines staffed by nurses), increases the opportunities for nurses to build on skills in telephone triage. These skills have already been used to good effect in out-of-hours services (Woodman, 1997; Lattimer *et al.*, 2000).

Early evaluation presents a mixed picture. Caller satisfaction rates have been high, but some caution has been expressed, particularly by the medical profession, who highlight the tension between: 'the often conflict-ing policy goals of consumer responsiveness and demand management' (Florin & Rosen, 1999, p. 5). The concern that Florin & Rosen express is that the existence of a 24-hour telephone service may paradoxically create increased demand for general practice, since many callers are referred to their GP. They argue that developing nurse triage through out-of-hours services or within general practice would ensure greater continuity of care whereas the 24-hour help line could concentrate on giving information.

Researchers using semi-structured interviews found that nurses undertak-ing telephone consultations developed skills to manage telephone consulta-tions, but these skills were developed in an ad hoc manner (Pettinari & Jessopp, 2001). The implications of these findings of development in practice pose a challenge for educators. They must first be aware of the developing know-ledge in practice and then bring that knowledge into academic settings for the benefit of future learners. As Buttigieg (1997, p. 70) states:

> What is required is a long-term vision and support from the statutory bodies to be innovative and flexible, to allow the production in a very short time of courses to meet service need. The pace of change means that many of the current education contracts are proving insufficiently flexible, and educationalists must be innovative if they are to meet the service demands.

A sound knowledge base and well documented competencies are prere-quisites for accountable practice. Recent changes in education have led to a competence-based approach. Since community nurses are required in future to take care of the wider community as well as individuals, they need to take cognisance of developing aspects of inter-agency care, with collaborative working and training being seen as central to future accountable practice (Buttigieg 1997; Thompson, 2001).

Recently there has been much improvement in the educational prepara-tion of practice nurses, with specific educational programmes for practice nurses and nurse practitioners (Reveley *et al.*, 2002), and the development and utilisation of protocols and guidelines requiring an annual review. As Saunders (2001) indicates, however, practice nurses need to ensure that they articulate their personal and professional requirements in their personal development plans and lobby hard for opportunities to remain responsive to changing health needs in the community.

Nurse prescribing

The extension of nurse prescribing with a wider drug formulary will sup-port the development of role expansion in the community (Walsh, 2001). Following Crown's review (Department of Health, 1999d), the recommen-dation to extend prescribing responsibilities to other groups of nurses and professionals has been accepted by the Government, so that it will no longer be confined to health visitors and district nurses. The range of ways in which nurses and others will prescribe for patients in their care includes supplementary prescribing, independent prescribing, and via patient group directives (Picton & Ganby, 2002). Supplementary prescribing is dependent on another's diagnosis and managed through an agreed clinical plan with the patient's permission.

Independent prescribing will occur when the prescriber takes responsibility and is accountable for the clinical assessment of the patient, which may include a diagnosis and any prescriptions issued. Group directives are written instructions designed for specific groups of patients who are not necessarily individually identified before presenting for treatment and who have specified clinical conditions. The evaluation of the introduction of prescribing by health visitors and district nurses found that nurse prescribing was effective, with a service much more appropriate and responsive to patient needs (Luker *et al.*, 1997).

The recent extension of prescribing has led to a refocusing of attention on the prerequisites of such a service by nurses and others such as pharmacists. As Picton & Ganby suggest, for nurses to exercise their duty of care appropriately they have to demonstrate their knowledge and competence on an ongoing basis, initially requiring access to an extended curriculum for education and training. This independence of nurse prescribing is underpinned by legislation. Therefore, nurses have to be aware of the additional legal accountability for practice when writing a prescription (Clarridge *et al.*, 2001; Picton & Ganby, 2002).

Picton & Ganby have developed a helpful competency framework for prescribing, which they suggest 'has the potential to be employed by individuals, teams or at an organisational level by using existing local infrastructures which may be in place to support continuing professional development' (Picton & Ganby, 2002, p. 93). Clarridge *et al.*, discussing district nursing, indicate the need to be mindful of resource implications when prescribing. This demonstrates accountability both to mangers and public resources but has to be balanced against assuring the most effective treatment for that individual client. This poses a potential conflict of accountability, one which medical colleagues have greater experience in managing. Clarridge *et al.* suggest that district nurses become involved in the developing collaborative prescribing partnerships within primary care, whether they be at practice, trust or LHCC level, to ensure successful integration of nurse prescribing.

Primary healthcare and public health nursing

There has been a resurgence of interest in the public health agenda in the UK, with policy strategies for public health from central and devolved governments (Department of Health Wales, 1998; Department of Health Scotland, 1998; Department of Health 1999d; Department of Health SSPS, 2000; Scottish Executive 2001b). For a considerable time public health objectives have been advocated by the WHO (WHO, 1986). It is evident that public health encompasses a much wider remit than just the medical model of health, and includes social and environmental aspects of health. Therefore, as Mason (2001) suggests, it is more meaningful to consider what is the contribution of nursing to the public health agenda since there need to be so many other agencies, for example housing, education, environmental health, transport and policing, involved in improving public health.

This challenge was taken up by the Scottish Executive Health Department (2001b) in its review of the contribution of nurses, midwives and health visitors to improving the public's health. Although acknowledging much good practice they indicate that contributions were often uncoordinated and ad hoc. They identified a lack of clear leadership and considered that nurses were not contributing significantly to strategy. The creation of a Public Health Institute has strengthened the opportunity to develop the skills of the workforce involved to contribute to the improvement of health, and also provides a forum for a leadership role for nurses alongside other professionals. Public health practitioners have been appointed to each LHCC. Their role includes clinical leadership, the collation of the wealth of knowledge that community practitioners have built up on the health status and needs of local communities, and mapping all local initiatives for improving public health (Scottish Executive Health Department, 2001b). These initiatives could also contribute to the accountability of nurses to their local communities in so far as the nurses have the position and the skills to articulate in a wider forum the obstacles that impede the choice of healthy options for individuals and families.

The public health agenda can also be seen as giving a welcome impetus to raising the profile of school nurses. As a service they have achieved lower professional status, with poorer educational opportunities, whilst traditionally employing a medical model in their work (Bines & Lightfoot, 1999). Bines & Lightfoot also showed that since school nurses' activities take place in education settings they can be marginalised and isolated from NHS colleagues. They highlight that as school nurses work with a captive audience, they are in an ideal position to make a contribution to young people's health. They also note, however, that school nurses have no authority, which means that they can not be accountable for carrying out health promotion work, since it is the school who has the formal responsibility for health education. Therefore, nurses must negotiate with schools to undertake health promotional work which may or may not be permitted by the school. In their research, Bines & Lightfoot found that schools often lacked an understanding of the role of the school nurse and they found that there was 'support for a framework, or "service level agreement" between individual schools and the local NHS trust for school services' (Bines & Lightfoot, 1999, p. 91) which could improve working relationships, facilitate joint planning for health promotion, and encourage a proactive response to needs (Department of Health, 1994b).

In the Scottish Executive's new model for practice:

> there is no discernable difference between the role of the health visitor and that of the school nurse, though the need for significant investment in the education of the school nursing force is recognised. In future both groups of nurses will be 'public health nurses', holding the same specialist practitioner qualification and sharing a joint education programme.
>
> (Scottish Executive Health Department, 2001, p. 29)

The potential for nurses in schools to contribute to current policy initiatives is high, but as Bines & Lightfoot (1999, p. 103) conclude: 'a clear role, based on evidence of need and capable of evaluation must be developed. This would contribute strongly to accountability in its various forms.' Perhaps one of the most important aspects of the public health agenda is a partnership approach to improving the health of communities. It is easy to argue that, although public health activity involves all nurses, health visitors in particular have a particular role to play as the principles of health visiting have their foundations in public health (CETHV, 1977; Twinn & Cowley, 1992).

Appleby & Sayer (2001), in considering the public health role of the health visitor, suggest examples of joint working involving tackling teenage pregnancy, mental health, Sure Start initiatives, domestic violence, or, for example, by improving nutritional health with dieticians, community workers, shopkeepers and local councillors. What this highlights is that the practitioner is accountable in various ways, e.g. in relation to external factors such as networking abilities, in the provision of knowledge and resources and maintaining relationships within the team, and in personal day-to-day relationships with individuals and families. As partnerships become increasingly formalised through, for example, the Joint Futures agenda which aims for greater integration of local services through joint resourcing and joint management of services with a single shared assessment (Scottish Executive Health Department, 2000b), it is imperative that the issues of accountability are addressed by working committees and steering groups. Multi-agency work requires that agreed roles, functions and lines of accountability are established, and that, in turn, requires an understanding of others' skills and expertise. Once again shared learning or secondments and attachments would facilitate understanding.

Relationships are at the heart of working in the community. Many community nurses are in the privileged position of being able to develop long-term partnerships with clients and families that can be used to enhance well-being for the whole family. De la Cuesta (1994) emphasises the need for developing trust as a basis for relationship-building, and Vehvilaeinen-Julkunen (1993) found, in research with public health nurses, that clients perceived the nurse as a helpful 'building block'. The ultimate aim of contacts with community nurses is to develop family self-help (Zerwekh, 1992). By building on trust, nurses work to develop family strength, uncovering the capabilities of that particular family. Zerwekh found that reinforcing the positive with mothers enhanced their self-esteem and empowered them to take charge of their lives.

The existence of a relationship does not in itself constitute partnership. That has to develop through the specific way that the nurse and client work and interact together (Gallant *et al.*, 2002). The nurse constantly has to find ways of sharing power and responsibility with clients. This working in partnership to foster empowerment, seen as part of developing practice with individuals, families and communities, is not without its pitfalls. Community nurses work within their professional framework, and health visitors, as well as helping families through empowerment, have to monitor families for any areas of concern. This is a dilemma for health visitors seeking to balance accountability to and advocacy for clients, accountability to management and the NMC. Zerwekh sees empowerment and enforcement as pulling in opposite directions, requiring community nurses to constantly balance loyalty to families and management.

Conclusion

Working in the community can bring enormous satisfaction for community nurses, and opportunities to foster and develop relationships with families and communities to establish partnerships with other agencies working to promote healthy communities. With the current focus on developing new ways of working in the community there are many opportunities for role development for community nurses, as well as the concomitant uncertainties. It is easy for individuals living through change to become inward looking and concerned for their own working conditions. Nurses, despite experiencing changes, must keep their focus on their clients. Issues of accountability, in all its guises, remain at the centre of practice.

Chapter 13

Clinical Governance, Accountability and Mental Health Nursing: an Emergent Story

Stephen Tilley

Introduction

I have argued previously that accountability is central to mental health nursing (Tilley, 1995). In this chapter I will construe accountability in the context provided by clinical governance. This new context accentuates the ambiguities and dilemmas inherent in mental health nursing conceived as accountable practice, ambiguities and dilemmas which I will interpret using Mishler's concepts of the 'voice of the lifeworld' and the 'voice of medicine' (Mishler, 1984). Under the auspices of clinical governance, will nurses in the ambit of clinical governance be reduced to scientific, bureaucratic deliverers of effective interventions (governed by the clinical), or will they develop a role in which they can enable the voice of the lifeworld to govern the clinical? The key issue is: how to govern the clinical. I will focus on these issues mainly with reference to UK policy and practice, but indicate also what we may learn from other countries' mental health policies (e.g. in New Zealand and in Ontario, Canada).

I will relate clinical governance and accountability to mental health nursing in two stages. First, while the fundamental elements of accountability in mental health nursing have carried forward into the clinical governance context, some aspects, for example justification by reference to policy or to the Nursing and Midwifery Council's *Code of Professional Conduct* (NMC, 2002b), are new. In addition, subsequent debates in the field of mental health nursing, related to clinical governance, deserve attention:

- debates over who determines the 'appropriate focus' of mental health nursing, and what that focus is
- debates over the roles of mental health nurses in 'control' as distinct from 'care', with reference to the new Scottish Mental Health Act

- tensions rooted in the 'Janus' nature of the nurse (accountable within an organisation ordered by clinical governance, and responsible to the person who is the patient)

Second, I will argue that mental health nurses can – and should – practise under the 'rule' of clinical governance only if that rule subordinates contractual obligations of 'clinical' accountability to primary covenantal obligations (of persons in relationship in community).

Review of themes from Tilley (1995)

The centrality of the topic

The analysis of accountability in Tilley (1995) can be extended in light of four developments:

- 'common accountability' and questions of governance are increasingly significant issues in public life
- accountability to managers is qualitatively different, as accountability for use of resources and for quality are conjoined
- professional accountability is problematic in new ways due in part to the emphasis on delivery of evidence-based interventions
- accountability of practitioners to researchers, and of researchers to practitioners, has likewise changed in the context of evidence-based practice

First, accountability is 'an aspect of the shared life which nurses and patients confront daily by virtue of participation in a society which increasingly stresses members' rights and obligations' (Tilley, 1995). Recognition, or assertion, of 'common demands for accountability' is heard more now than in 1994, in discourses on rights and obligations. Prime Minister Blair's New Labour Government has increasingly stressed the balance of rights and obligations, raising the prospect that rights to appropriate services might be forfeit if users fail to meet obligations of involvement in planning and evaluation (Thompson & Clare, 2002). Thus we face an increasingly clear imperative of reflexivity in discussions of accountability: we shape the society in the context of which we consider accountability and clinical governance, and are shaped by it. Our very identities (as I, we, or you), as users of services as well as professionals, must be equally reflexive.

Second, my 1995 comment that 'psychiatric nurses, being employed in institutions, are accountable to their managers' now requires re-contextualisation in light of the development of clinical governance. This aspect is addressed further below.

Third, references to the UKCC code of practice and UKCC and RCN documents on accountability need to be updated. Or do they? A notable feature of the culture of accountability and clinical governance is that it occasions anxiety, not least by stimulating us to ask 'is my knowledge/

understanding of X up-to-date?' The Nursing and Midwifery Council's *Code of Professional Conduct* (NMC, 2002b) states that:

> You are accountable for your practice. This means that you are answerable for your actions and omissions, regardless of advice or directions from another professional. (p. 3)

> You are personally accountable for ensuring that you promote and protect the interests and dignity of patients and clients, irrespective of gender, age, race, ability, sexuality, economic status, lifestyle, culture and religious or political belief. (p. 4)

Noteworthy is the NMC's statement that:

> As a registered nurse or midwife, you must maintain your professional knowledge and competence. . . . You have a responsibility to deliver care based on current evidence, best practice and, where applicable, validated research when it is available. (p. 8)

The NMC guidelines thus bring the metaphor of 'service delivery' into 'top-down' discourses on/of nursing accountability.[1] 'Practice' is interpreted as 'delivery of evidence-based care'.

These statements beg a number of questions, e.g. 'Is care something that is delivered?' and 'Are professionals (essentially) deliverers of care?' 'Delivery' implies that what is delivered is conveyed in some way from one place to another; a deliverer and a receiver. Is care in mental health nursing like this? Ryan *et al.* (1998) summarised the argument that the person who is mentally ill contributes to the meaning of what is done in care, and this theme is developed in more recent literature on 'recovery'. Barker (1989) elaborated 'care' as 'trephotaxis,' creation of the appropriate conditions for growth and development. The creation of conditions, or affordances (Shotter, 1984) is not a matter of delivery of something to someone or someplace. Nor can the professional be construed as a 'deliverer', unless in the shape of Socrates' 'midwife'.

Fourth, the view that 'psychiatric nurses may be accountable to researchers or professionalisers' (Tilley, 1995) also bears revisiting. Over the past ten years, mental health nursing research, and arguments about research, have developed rapidly. The Commentary section of the *Journal of Psychiatric and Mental Health Nursing* has been a particularly 'hot' site for debates about mental health nursing research, its role in relation to professionalisation, and its relevance to practice. The 1996 and 2001 Research Assessment Exercises have occasioned debates about the basis on which mental health

---

[1] Newell, a nursing professor and advocate of evidence-based practice, was quoted as saying: 'We would do well to get away from the notion of professionals as experts about patients' lives. Professionals are experts about the delivery of care. Therefore we should confine ourselves to that area of expertise.' (Newell, cited in Cole & Oxtoby, 2002).

nurse researchers can be called to account by their academic and practice 'peers'.

Accounts

Further consideration of 'accounts' is warranted in light of the advancing ideology of evidence-based practice, disputes about the auspices of accounts, e.g. based on nursing theory or on biomedical theories of schizophrenia[2], and arguments about the adequacy of accounts appealing to common sense rather than theory[3].

The sections on 'Paradigm and template accounts' and on 'Accounts and working ideologies' (Tilley, 1995), too, bear reconsideration. Under 'a shift in meaning of accounts' I noted that from an interpretive perspective 'accounts are regarded as discursive events which interpret the situation and order action within it'. Clinical governance constitutes a kind of 'general account' ordering trusts' accounting practices – for both quality and finance – so that the executive and board are accountable for both. Two spheres, before distinct, are now conjoined and co-ordered. I will argue below, however, that this conjoining is problematic to the extent that one of the dimensions – quality – resists structuring in this way.

Clinical governance is a working ideology, with a central claim, that the quality of work in the trust can be construed in terms of 'delivery' of 'interventions' justified by reference to an evidence-base. The power of this paradigm account extends beyond trusts and the clinical sphere. It is central also to the working ideology of nursing educational providers, whose practices are increasingly geared into those of service providers (perhaps more in service agreements in England, Wales and Northern Ireland than in Scotland). To the extent that trusts require staff to be fit for practice regulated by clinical governance, education providers aim to demonstrate their *own* 'fitness for purpose' by preparing students to construct service paradigm-shaped accounts.

---

[2] See, for example, disputes between Kevin Gournay, Phil Barker and others (Gournay, 1995; Barker & Reynolds, 1996; Rolfe, 1996; Gournay, 1996; Dawson, 1997; Gournay, 1997) about the status of nursing theories and models, and theories of schizophrenia.

[3] With regard to 'accounts, common sense and professional judgement' I have revised my views on the adequacy of Annie Altschul's arguments about nurses' justification of their accounts by appeal to 'common sense' rather than a theory or an 'identifiable perspective'. Altschul clarified the basis of her argument: 'I am not against common sense. But my job was to teach students, and common sense is not something that can be taught' (Altschul, 1999). In writing thus, Annie was not (as I had construed her) standing *outside* the situation of practice, holding up a template of theoretical knowledge and noting only 'absence'. Rather, she was speaking from her primary standpoint as *teacher* (of professional nurses) articulating the epistemological and ethical base from which she addressed and constituted her community. From her perspective, if common sense sufficed for practice, *she* could not practise accountably as a teacher. As teacher, she could not let the nurse in practice (or me as researcher) rest with the implication of failure to offer an account beyond 'it's common sense'.

The quality of debate in the field of psychiatric and mental health nursing has improved substantially over the past ten years, and challenges to the dominant 'paradigm account' are more fully developed than they were in 1995.[4] The best UK example of a rival paradigm is the Tidal Model promulgated by Phil Barker and colleagues (Barker, 2001). A key element of the 'working ideology' of that model is the co-construction, by nurse and the person/patient, of a narrative of problems and responses aimed at recovery of mental health.[5]

Accounting

I noted (Tilley, 1995) that 'accounts are structured in systems and processes of accounting.' Clearly, clinical governance implies and establishes such systems and processes. The 'something to be accounted for' is quality, and the 'somebody [who] has an interest in that something' is ultimately the chief executive or trust board. I have noted above some issues related to definition of quality, in this context. 'Accounting [as] a form of labour', and the related notions of the 'value of labour' bear further consideration. For example, if systems of accounting do not allow for, or prevent, conveying the person/patient's 'story' and its relevance for care, the value of labour done under the auspices of a model in which that labour is essential, would be less (Barker, 2002).

To a greater extent than in 1995, formal systems of accounting are computer-based, and may entail construction of integrated records. The use of such records may in turn be related to aims to provide integrated care, itself a hallmark of quality of care and of the service. Here it is important to consider the role of informal accounting, that is, the accounting that accompanies practice and use of records but is not documented. Precisely to the extent that accounting systems and related hardware and software offer the promise of representing the quality of care (here, integration), they also pose the problem of how to tolerate the inevitable incompleteness of the representation. Any member of the organisation might have interests in maintaining omissions from the record, and in resisting the system's (intended or unintended) power effects. Members of different professions, e.g. social work and nursing, may think a patient/person's interests better served (or care better achieved) by keeping some information off the record. New systems of accounting pose new problems and obligations of resistance.

---

[4]   See for example debates in the *Journal of Psychiatric and Mental Health Nursing* on the value of nursing models (see footnote 3, above). See also justifications of the 'Thorn Programme' courses (e.g. Gournay, 1995) as exemplifying an educational paradigm account shaped for fit with clinical governance-driven service providers.
[5]   Metaphor and narrative are also promoted as forms *particularly* appropriate for accounting for work under the auspices of 'recovery' in work in New Zealand (Mental Health Commission, 1998, 2002).

Accountability

As noted in Tilley (1995), analysis of accountability requires attention to the relationship between accounts, accounting and accountability:

> If accounts relate more to knowledge, and accounting to systems of power, accountability relates to moral order. Accounts are devices for, and occasions for, discipline; opening one to surveillance, to judgement of normality, to interpretation and to correction. Accounting is a form of discipline – a process of confession and response. Accountability refers to the rights and obligations entailed by participation in a system of accounts and the norms related to the system of accounting. It involves taking one's place in a system of accounting, becoming the 'I' in documents circulated to 'them'.
>
> The counterpart to formal and informal accounts and systems of accounting is formal and informal accountability. Nurses as accountable practitioners can be considered 'Janus-faced'. Janus, the deity associated with openings, is an apt emblem for nurses who have to keep patients 'open' as accountable subjects in wards or in the community; to keep open the possibilities of exchange between hospital and community; to act as gatekeepers in systems of need and resource determination. Janus had two faces: one facing in, the other out. Psychiatric nurses are accountable to the wider community of which they and patients are members, the community knit together by common sense. They are also accountable to professional and institutional bodies requiring them to be ready and willing to provide accounts legitimated by reference to law, theory, codes of conduct or procedure manuals. Janus-faced accountability – implying accountability to managers and the profession, as well as responsibility to the patient in face-to-face interaction Ryan[6] – is for practical purposes the essential characteristic of psychiatric nursing.   (Tilley, 1995)

This analysis holds in the context of clinical governance, but requires elaboration. The problematic of the Janus-faced nurse has changed. Accountability to the 'institutional body' under the auspices of clinical governance means accountability to the trust chief executive (to enable the chief executive to be accountable) for both financial matters and quality. Or rather, it means accountability to the chief executive for the quality of 'clinical' care (in the form of 'deliverable' interventions). Janus facing this way exercises a highly *role-bound* accountability, not a *person-based* responsibility. But facing the person who is a patient, Janus practises care as a 'person art' (Ryan, 1985), not delivering, but co-developing. To the extent that clinical governance manages to reduce care to clinical dimensions, it reduces the capa-

---

[6]   Ryan, D. (1993) 'Ambiguity in Nursing'. Seminar given to Department of Nursing Studies, University of Edinburgh, Edinburgh.

city of the person-nurse to fulfil her or his essential *professional* remit: to use the resources of the institution (hospital, other institution, or community-based) to meet the obligations of care mandated by the person-patient. For Janus <u>thus</u> faced, the person-patient 'remains the source of authority which underpins that care' (Ryan, 1997). The person-patient's authority cannot be co-opted into a system of clinical governance.

The reader may well question whether that last statement can stand, given mental health nurses' roles in 'control of' as well as 'care of' people with mental health problems. Indeed, the patient's authority might be seen as co-opted in two ways. First, despite requirements of user involvement in mental health care and services (SOHD, 1997), some mechanisms for achieving this in effect co-opt users by offering themselves in the role of relatively weak and passive forms of 'involvement'. Second, patients detained under the terms of the Mental Health (Scotland) Act 1984 might be seen as having their authority co-opted for the period in which they are determined to be not responsible for their actions or decision. Following an extensive consultation process in Scotland the Millan Report (Scottish Executive Health Department, 2001a) highlighted a number of 'changes in mental health care' as partial justification for proposing a new Act. These include:

- the growth in recognition of the rights of service users to greater involvement in decisions concerning them
- increasing interest in . . . 'contracts for care' or advance statements, which allow people to set out, when well, the care they would wish to receive should they become unwell
- development of the concept of 'reciprocity': that society owes some duty to provide appropriate services to those who have been required to accept treatment against their will
  (Scottish Executive Health Department, 2001a, pp. 3–5)

The source of authority underpinning care, for those detained or treated against their will, remains obscure. While some patient/persons might mandate in advance what they want done by professionals and others when they are not competent (e.g. with advance directives), those who do not might well be seen, and see themselves, as having their authority co-opted if 'sectioned' under the Act. The Millan Report sets out a number of principles intended to guide mental health nurses' deliberations on their responsibilities as persons and professionals, in managing accountability when control is a central issue. These are justice (non-discrimination, equality, respect for diversity, reciprocity); autonomy (informal care, participation, respect for carers); beneficence and non-maleficence (least restrictive alternative, benefit, child welfare) (Scottish Executive Health Department, 2001a, pp. 18–21). Taken together, these principles indicate attention to the relationships of persons and citizens, in light of which the Act is to be interpreted and used in practice. They point to wider contexts of political and social governance relevant to justification of clinical practice.

Accountability and clinical governance

This review has indicated key issues relating to accounts, accounting and accountability in the context of clinical governance. I now turn to argue that clinical governance – the policy, and the set of practices in which that policy is realised – is problematic, to the extent that it stresses accountability for clinical matters at the expense of attention to the more fundamental contexts of accountability implied by governance, and to the extent that it promotes the 'voice of medicine' over the 'voice of the lifeworld' and 'effectiveness' over 'humane care' as the basis of relationships in healthcare (Mishler, 1984).

The voice of medicine expresses 'the biomedical model as the perspective within which the patients' statements are interpreted [which] allows the 'medical' tasks of diagnosis and prescription' (Mishler, 1984, p. 63). By contrast:

> The voice of the lifeworld refers to the patient's contextually-grounded experiences of events and problems in her life . . . expressed from the perspective of a 'natural attitude'. . . . In contrast, the voice of medicine reflects a technical interest and expresses a 'scientific attitude'. The meaning of events is provided through abstract rules that serve to decontextualise events, to remove them from particular personal and social context.
>
> (Mishler, 1984, p. 104)

The 'weight' to be accorded the voice of medicine, in relation to the voice of the lifeworld, was not specified when clinical governance was introduced. Indeed, according to Miller's (2001, p. 1) account, clinical governance was underspecified, appearing as something 'almost hidden away':

> The publication of the NHS White Paper, *Designed to Care* (Scottish Executive Health Department, 1998), heralded a number of significant changes to the structure of the NHS in Scotland. . . . Almost hidden away in paragraph 68 were two words – clinical governance – that appear to have had a much greater impact on the health service than any of the structure changes.

Nonetheless, the power of the voice of medicine was implied in an essentially modernist[7] system of accountability:

---

[7] A key theme in modernism is division of labour and specification of role. The Government constructs higher education institutions (HEIs) as 'partners' with the local NHS trusts in promoting the NHS modernisation agenda. Researchers in HEIs are constructed as producers of the evidence to be fed into practice to modernise the health service; teachers as deliverers of evidence-based knowledge suitable for consumption by students. Healthcare workers including mental health nurses are constructed as deliverers of evidence-based interventions. Educational governance gears into clinical governance (e.g. through the process of HEIs contracting through local workforce confederations to provide education determined by service providers' definition of 'fitness for purpose'). Both gear into the Government's 'NHS modernising' agenda.

Clinical governance . . . is a framework that provides the means by which organisations ensure the provision of high quality clinical care by making individuals accountable for setting, maintaining and monitoring performance standards. (Miller, 2001, pp. 2–3)

'Clinical', 'performance', 'standards', 'making accountable', 'individuals' are ingredients in a modernist recipe, with the key term 'accountability':

It could be argued that the Conservative Government of 1989 placed an emphasis on value for money and market ideals whereas the Labour Government of 1997 placed emphasis on quality and public service ideals. . . . Responsibility and accountability for quality of care were less explicit [in the 1989 White Paper], and it is reasonable to conclude that the main difference of the new arrangement relates to the exercising of accountability. (Miller, 2001, p. 2)

Thus, 'hidden' in the policy announcing clinical governance was a more powerful form of professional accountability grounded in the voice of medicine. Where the voice of the lifeworld appeared, it was in the context of assuring effectiveness: 'Clinical governance is everybody's business. . . . User/patient involvement: the involvement of patients and the wider public is essential to effective clinical governance (Miller, 2001, pp. 9, 4).

The reader may find the prospect sketched above unlikely, a caricature of clinical governance, and counter that the thrust of clinical governance is that healthcare workers should use evidence to provide good quality care, and that one dimension of quality is that it is person-focused. 'Evidence-based practice' means using the best available evidence to provide care of benefit to particular persons in particular contexts. There is, according to this account, little to fear from clinical governance, seen as a means of regulating and assuring 'deliverance' of quality care.

In support of this response one might cite Sir David Goldberg's foreword to Newell & Gournay's *Mental Health Nursing: An Evidence-based Approach*:

Evidence-based medicine may well be the ultimate goal, but we may need to ask ourselves what the *patient-based evidence* is for a particular line of treatment, and to reconcile ourselves to the fact that we sometimes have no alternative but to rely on 'established wisdom'. (Goldberg, 2000)

However, 'reconcile' and 'no alternative' suggest a medical voice overshadowing that of the lifeworld; established wisdom residual to 'evidence-based medicine'.

We can heuristically contrast Goldberg's view with that of the 'father' of the evidence-based practice movement, Archie Cochrane. Grounds for a different account of the 'order' of the voices of medicine and the lifeworld can be found in an excerpt from Cochrane's autobiography relating his experience as a medical officer in a World War II prisoner of war camp:

Another event at Elsterhorst had a marked effect on me. The Germans dumped a young Soviet prisoner in my ward late one night. The ward was full, so I put him in my room as he was moribund and screaming and I did not want to wake the ward. I examined him. He had obvious gross bilateral cavitation and a severe pleural rub. I thought the latter was the cause of the pain and the screaming. I had no morphia, just aspirin, which had no effect. I felt desperate. I knew very little Russian then and there was no one in the ward who did. I finally instinctively sat down on the bed and took him in my arms, and the screaming stopped almost at once. He died peacefully in my arms a few hours later. It was not the pleurisy that caused the screaming but loneliness. It was a wonderful education about the care of the dying. I was ashamed of my misdiagnosis and kept the story secret.

(Cochrane, 1989)

Two aspects of this story are noteworthy. First, Cochrane's arms remind us that the individual practitioner is 'the nearest hand in a chain of caring hands held out to overcome anguish' (Ryan, 1997, p. 121). 'Evidenced' in Cochrane's account is the intuitive member of a *culture* which recognises persons, and which values human caring responses to suffering. This knowledge is neither 'individual' nor 'clinical'. Anyone sufficiently informed by humane care might have done, intuitively, what Cochrane did. Saying this does not diminish the epistemological value of decontextualising, bias-reducing clinical knowledge. Cochrane's secret story conveys our common obligation to respond to our fellow humans who suffer illness or aspire to health with the full range of responses grounded in traditions of caring practice, including (but not privileging) the 'clinical'. The real value of the 'clinical' (and its relevant epistemology) is seen by setting it in relation to something of greater value. The clinical is governed here by setting it wider cultural and values contexts.

One lesson of Cochrane's once-secret story is thus that the meaning we attribute to clinical governance depends on how we contextualise it in relation to deeper grounds of governance: the basis of our relationships in political and social contexts. The larger text in relation to which we should read clinical governance should be a culture in which each holds all to account for how we develop and use clinical knowledge to promote the growth and development of persons in relationship in community.

Second, we note that Cochrane kept the 'right diagnosis' 'hidden'; kept himself from the gaze of accountability by not telling (or rather, deferring telling) his story. Publication of the voice of the lifeworld was withheld. Withheld too was the implication of a hierarchy of diagnoses: of those diseases located *in* the patient as an object of medical knowledge, and those 'diseases' located in the relationship *between* the patient as a person and the persons responding to his or her suffering. Cochrane's 'hiding' of his story signifies that there was insufficient scope in the language game of medicine (and healthcare more generally) to speak about the values base, and the fuller range of human caring responses, actually relevant to care.

The role of the mental health nurse in clinical governance

It is clear, then, that we now face a primary question: does clinical governance provide greater scope for stories like the one Cochrane hid? Does it project the voice of the lifeworld, as well as the voice of medicine, and set both in the context of the wider culture sustaining health and healthcare?

Mental health nursing literature has not adequately resolved the tensions imposed by mental health nurses' dual obligations as both whole persons/members of community and agencies of effective intervention. Writers increasingly propose versions of both and solutions to practising in light of those tensions (e.g. Repper, 2000). Some, however, emphasise one register over the other. Thus Newell & Gournay see three interrelated needs:

- a 'need within mental health nursing . . . for appropriate evidence upon which to base our clinical practice as nurses'
- a need to participate in research and practice in multidisciplinary teams
- a need, to 'have a coherent, authoritative voice within the discipline of mental healthcare . . . through participation in the National Health Service's evidence-based practice, clinical effectiveness, and clinical governance agendas'   (Newell & Gournay, 2000)

While some contributors to their text speak more obviously in the voice of the lifeworld (e.g. Campbell, 2000), the hierarchy-of-evidence warrants are those associated with the voice of medicine (see the quotation from Goldberg, above). More recently, Gournay (2003) notes the continuing 'need to emphasise a starting point for everyone involved in health services research to listen to what users have to say about what is important to them', and that: 'although this rhetoric has been sounded for more than a decade . . . true central consumer involvement in health services research is still a dream' (Gournay, 2003, p. 248). Gournay follows this claim for the value of the consumer's view with an assertion that 'mental health nursing is poorly served by its academic infrastructure' and that:

> very few professors of mental health nursing have any formal training in health services research methods and most are largely ignorant of basic topics such as epidemiology, quantitative methodologies and the realistic application of power calculations for the purposes of determining reasonable sample sizes.   (Gournay, 2003, p. 249)

How emphasis on these methodologies (and the implied hierarchy of evidence) squares with giving priority to 'what users have to say is important to them' is not addressed. By contrast, Barker's account of the Tidal Model as a 'discrete' nursing contribution to 'a multidisciplinary care and treatment process' (Barker, 2001, p. 234) warrants a narrative-based methodology in terms redolent of the lifeworld. In giving precedence to the person's story the Tidal Model acknowledges that the narrative is the location for the person's enactment of life (p. 236).

Barker stresses the need to avoid 'stifling the continued search for true under-standing of . . . problems of human living' (p. 233), and to promote instead a 'human living' approach grounded in nursing's 'longstanding attachment to the concept of caring through interpersonal relationships' (p. 237).

We can hear in these texts mental health nursing versions of the voice of medicine and the voice of the lifeworld[8], and of the corresponding criteria for judging the adequacy of care: effectiveness and humaneness (Mishler, 1984, p. 63). What is at stake is the possibility of what Mishler called 'humane care':

> A serious problem arises when these two criteria, humaneness and effect-iveness, are placed in opposition. . . . [Humane] care is effective care and, to be effective care must be humane. . . . [Humane] care refers to the primacy accorded to patients' lifeworld contexts of meaning as the basis for understanding, diagnosing, and treating their problems. . . . A discourse dominated by the voice of medicine represents a practice that is not humane . . . such a practice is also an ineffective practice.
>
> (Mishler, 1984, pp. 191–2)

He argues further that 'strengthening the voice of the lifeworld promotes both humaneness and effectiveness of care', and that:

> Given that current forms of clinical practice are based on and incorpor-ate an asymmetical power relationship between patients and healthcare workers . . . achieving humane care is dependent upon empowering patients.   (Mishler, 1984; p. 193)

Following Mishler's argument, we can draw implications for mental health nurses in the context of clinical governance sketched in this chapter. Nurses should resist participation in a clinical governance language game ruled by the 'delivery of interventions' metaphor; resist reduction to the role of deliverers of effective interventions. Obligations to fulfil contracts to 'deliver' effective care are subordinate to the covenantal obligation to sustain the person who is ill in his or her participation in community.[9]

As individuals, mental health nurses have limited capacity to order the voices of medicine and the lifeworld appropriately, and to manage the tensions of practice for the benefit of those persons/patients with whom they have obligations of both covenant and contract. They could be empowered to do so if policy, at trust and national level, articulated more clearly the values base for mental health care grounded in the voice of the lifeworld and the voice of medicine rightly ordered.

Assertive policies, addressing the relationship between the voice of the life-world and the voice of medicine, have been put into practice in New Zealand

---

[8] I note the contrast, but also that both Gournay and Barker have acknowledged the rela-tive value of the respective 'other' voice.
[9] For elaboration on the contract/covenant distinction see Tilley & Pollock (1999).

and in Ontario, Canada. The *New Framework for Support* (Trainor *et al.*, 1999) in Ontario proposes reconceptualisation of mental health and illness, based on a 'balanced knowledge base' incorporating medical/clinical, social science, experiential, and customary traditional knowledge. It provides a model of how to order clinical knowledge in a wider context of knowledge governance. Both the Ontario *Framework* and the New Zealand *Blueprint for Mental Health* (Mental Health Commission, 1998; cf. Mental Health Commission, 2002) promote 'recovery' as a central principle. The *New Framework* cites Anthony's definition of 'recovery':

> Recovery is described as a deeply personal, unique process of changing one's attitudes, values, feelings, goals, skills, and/or roles. It is a way of living a satisfying, hopeful, and contributing life even with limitations caused by an illness. Recovery involves the development of new meaning and purpose in one's life as one grows beyond the catastrophic effects of mental illness.
>
> Recovery from mental illness involves much more than recovery from the illness itself. People with mental illness may have to recover from the stigma they have incorporated into their very being; from the iatrogenic effects of treatment settings; from lack of recent opportunities for self-determination; from the negative side effects of unemployment; and from crushed dreams. (Anthony, 1993, p. 15)

We can learn from these models as we seek, in both practice and policy, to realise the significance of clinical governance, and the contemporary implications of Cochrane's secret story. Necessarily amphibians[10] as we participate in systems of accountability and clinical governance, we are called to order and integrate two voices, two modes of caring. We can do so more effectively, in the interests of humane care, if able to justify our practice by reference to trust and national policies on clinical governance. These policies should set our effectiveness-directed, contract-mediated clinical roles in the context of covenantal, persons-in-relationship-in-community-grounded governance. The emerging story of humane care can best develop if policy enriches the language game, and furnishes a more congenial 'dwelling' for those who participate in systems of clinical accountability for mental health care, and human relations.

---

[10] This account poses a different role for the clinical governance-environment version of the 'amphibian' nurse described by Ryan (1997) and sketched in Tilley (1995). In this version, we amphibians must now embody the tensions of the coexistence of modernity and its antithesis; with the general manager logically the Big Amphibian incorporating the tensions of all in the trust, to fulfil his/her responsibility of ensuring the quality of covenant while delivering on contract. See also Ryan & Mowat (2003).

Chapter 14

Accountability in Nursing Research

Alison Tierney and Roger Watson

Introduction

Most of the discussion and the literature relating to accountability referred to in this book is centred on nursing practice. The matter of accountability in the field of nursing research has not been written about much (Tierney, 1995). This does not mean, of course, that nurse researchers have not been accountable: like many researchers, especially those whose work involves vulnerable people, nurse researchers have multiple accountabilities to address. In recent years the issue of accountability in health and social care research has been brought into sharp focus. Specifically, the UK's Departments of Health have introduced a framework for the governance of research in health and social care (Department of Health, 2001f). The accountability of nurse researchers can be reconsidered in this light. Before doing so, however, we start this chapter by considering research as a responsibility of an accountable profession.

Research as a responsibility of an accountable profession

If nurses are to be truly accountable for their practice then they must accept responsibility for advancing the knowledge base of nursing and, therefore, to engage with research. It was a significant turning point in the UK when the Briggs Committee recommended that 'nursing should become a research-based profession' and declared that 'a sense of the need for research should become a part of the mental equipment of every practising nurse' (HMSO, 1972). At that time – the early 1970s – the amount of research activity in nursing was very limited, at least, outside North America. Few nurses had undergone formal research training or accumulated research experience. The nursing curriculum paid scant attention to research and nursing students could reach registration without having been introduced to research. At the same time, nurses in practice were either unconcerned about research or frankly hostile to the introduction of an apparently unnecessary 'academic' pursuit in a practical profession.

Times have changed. Although not all nurses are positive about research, there cannot be a nursing student nowadays who has not been exposed to research and, over the past five years or so, 'evidence-based practice' has become a well understood tenet in nursing (Thompson, 2001).

Therefore, over a comparatively short timespan, and with relatively limited resources, the extent of research development in nursing is nothing other than impressive (Robinson *et al.*, 2002). But it is equally important for the profession to acknowledge that its research capability is weak, and that ongoing strategic development of research in nursing remains essential. The *Strategy for Research in Nursing, Midwifery and Health Visiting*, which was formulated by a task force on behalf of the UK Government in 1993 (Department of Health, 1993b) represented an important early step forward in that direction.

More recently, the need for further, concerted effort to boost research capacity and activity in the nursing profession has been highlighted in *Making a Difference* (Department of Health, 1999e) and, in Scotland, the formulation of a comprehensive *Nursing and Midwifery Research and Development Strategy* (Scottish Executive Health Department, 2002) signals the beginning of truly concerted action at all levels. There is clear recognition now that there are not enough nurses with research training and experience, and compared with many other professions, nursing has fewer doctoral students (Higher Education Funding Council for England, 2001). Steps are being taken to address this, not only by the UK Government (Department of Health, 2000a) but also by organisations such as the Health Foundation (PPP Foundation) and the Smith & Nephew Foundation, which have initiated research training schemes for nurses and allied health professions, in response to the need.

Even if capacity is increased, however, it is also the case that there are few funds earmarked specifically for nursing research in the UK, and no dedicated research council. Over 100 medical charities were asked about whether or not they would fund nursing research, but few indicated that they would do so (Crofts & McMahon, 2000). The Government continues to recognise the contribution that research has to make to healthcare and although the vast majority of funds are still aimed at supporting basic medical research there is increasing support for applied research relating to service delivery and organisation and, being more concerned with patient needs and priorities, research in this area is more applicable to nursing (Department of Health, 2000a).

There are still many barriers to research in nursing but, on the whole, progress over the past decade has been considerable, not only in the UK but also in most other European countries and, indeed, across the world.

Accountability in nursing research

Having considered research as a responsibility of an accountable profession, the remainder of this chapter will consider accountability in nursing research in terms of the personal accountability of nurses whose sole or primary occupation is research. Most of what is said, however, will have relevance for any nurse who is directly or indirectly involved in research even although not a career researcher.

Nurse researchers as nurses

The *Code of Professional Conduct* (NMC, 2002b) has the purpose of informing 'the professions of the standard of professional conduct required of them in the exercise of their professional accountability and practice'. The code is as pertinent to nursing research as to any other area of professional nursing.

The code goes on to say that as a registered nurse or midwife 'you are personally accountable for your practice'. Again, this statement is as applicable to a nurse researcher as to any nurse. Although the ensuing specifications in the code regarding the exercise of professional accountability were apparently written with practising nurses in mind, each has direct or indirect relevance for nurse researchers. Indeed, many seem particularly pertinent: for example, those that refer to the primacy of patients' interests and well-being; consent to treatment; confidentiality and minimising risk.

The importance of accountability in research

The concept of accountability has self-evident importance in research. *The Oxford Reference Dictionary* defines 'accountable' as 'having to account (for one's actions)'; 'to account for' as 'to give a reckoning of'; and 'an account' as 'a description, a report'. It is clear, therefore, that accountability is an important, integral aspect of research and so it is rather surprising that it has been so neglected in the research literature and in the literature on professional accountability. Perhaps accountability in research has simply been taken for granted, and its exercise in practice regarded as nothing other than straightforward.

This lack of attention is not peculiar to nursing. The issue of accountability in research in any field rarely seems to have been a routine matter of public or professional debate. Questions of accountability in research really only come to the fore when a case of academic fraud or financial indiscretion in the use of research funds is exposed. What these cases tend to reveal is the high degree of autonomy that scientists tend to enjoy, and the extent to which their work is conducted without interference. It has been rare for researchers to be publicly called to account for the conduct and results of their research. This, however, has been changing and the existence of fraud in scientific research is well publicised with numerous examples of specific incidents which are often highlighted by editors of journals.

In spite of this increasing scrutiny of research, most researchers continue to work with a high degree of autonomy. The other side of this coin, then, is that researchers must accept a high degree of personal responsibility for the quality and integrity of their work, and for the proper use of research funds. With personal responsibility comes individual accountability. Indeed the researcher's final account in the form of research publications becomes available for open critical appraisal, not only by experts and peers, but also by the wider public through the lay media. If a researcher's account is found wanting, at best further grants will be hard or impossible to obtain, and at worst there will be no further career prospects in research. In scandalous cases there may even be public disgrace or prosecution. The framework for research governance (Department of Health, 2001f) introduced recently in the UK – as already mentioned – is designed to avoid the problems arising from poorly managed or badly conducted research in the fields of health and social care. This will be considered later in the chapter.

In comparison with 'high science', the world of nursing research to date has concerned only modest amounts of money and with issues which have rarely been seen as highly controversial. Hence, there has been no great public or professional concern about the standards or regulation of nursing research. To our knowledge, no nurse has been struck off the register for improprieties in the course of research. Except for large-scale projects, or programmes which are government-funded, the outputs of research in nursing have not been subjected to the degree of scrutiny and criticism that is more commonplace in other disciplines.

The greater external interest in, and scrutiny of, nursing research in the UK has come about through the Research Assessment Exercise (RAE), although outside the higher education sector, the implications of the RAE have not made any great impact across – and beyond – the nursing profession. The fact that the discipline of nursing has come 'bottom of the RAE league table', however, has raised questions in some quarters about current standards of nursing research (Robinson *et al.*, 2002). Equally, it could be argued that health research funders should be held accountable for their inadequate support of nursing research over past decades.

We move now from discussion of what aspects of accountability are important for nursing research to specific issues attributed to the accountability of individual nurse researchers in the course of conducting research.

To whom are nurse researchers accountable?

By definition, accountability is to another party or parties, including those in positions of authority, but also to those who are in positions of equality and dependence. Accountability to those in positions of authority arises from the notion of 'dueness', whereas the idea of 'duty' is connected with accountability to those in equal or dependent positions. Both of these terms – dueness and duty – are linked with the concept of accountability, and both apply in the context of research. Within the current framework for research

Table 14.1   The people and organisations involved
in health or social care research (adapted from
Department of Health 2001f).

Participants
Researchers
Principal investigator
Funder(s)
Sponsor
Employing organisation(s)
Care organisation
Responsible care professional
Research ethics committee

---

governance Table 14.1 shows who the different parties involved in research
are. These will be referred to below.

In the field of practice, nurses are accountable to their clients, the profession,
their manager and their employing organisation, as well as to themselves,
according to Evans (1993). The same sort of mix applies in the field of research.
Accountability in the case of nurse researchers will be examined in relation
to the sponsor (the grant-giving body); research ethics committees (the main
purpose of which is to protect the public); research participants; those who
control research access (the 'gatekeepers'); co-researchers; the profession
(the primary consumers of nursing research); and, finally, the wider public.

Accountability to the sponsor

For any researcher, the most formal line of accountability is usually to the
sponsor. Indeed, ensuring that a research project is adequately financed from
the outset is a prime responsibility of an accountable researcher. This principle applies irrespective of the size of the project: all research costs money.
There are always labour costs and, even in the most modest of projects, there
will be at least some material costs as well. Even the smallest of research
projects needs a budget, therefore, and this in turn requires a sponsor. This
is one aspect of health and social research which has been tightened up considerably in the UK with the advent of research governance (Department of
Health, 2001f).

Who are the sponsors?
Sponsorship for a nursing research study can be sought from a wide range
of sources. Government funding is a major source of finance for studies in
nursing and healthcare. In the UK, research funding for such studies is dis-
bursed through the Research and Development section of the Department

of Health in England or equivalent offices in the other three countries of the UK. Awards are made on the basis of peer review of research grant applications and committee agreement in line with the sponsor's priorities. The NHS itself has a budget for research and development and all staff working in the NHS, nurses included, can apply for these research funds. Beyond Government and the NHS, funding for research in the field of healthcare is available from a host of charitable trusts as well as from the commercial sector, including pharmaceutical companies and other suppliers. Research funding is available; the challenge is for nurses to become more successful at accessing it. The Royal College of Nursing Research & Development Coordinating Centre (www.man.ac.uk/rcn) provides information on research activity in the UK and opportunities for funding.

How is accountability to sponsors defined?

Irrespective of the source or amount of funding, all sponsors enter into some form of contractual relationship with the researcher. The researcher may be expected to be directly accountable to the sponsor, or the line of accountability may be through an intermediary, for example, the head of department in the case of a nurse researcher based in a university, or a general manager or clinical director or research and development director in the case of a nurse who is an NHS employee. These more senior members of the organisation concerned may be formally appointed by the sponsor as the grant-holder and, in such cases, they are the people to whom the researcher is accountable on a day-to-day basis, and through them to the sponsor. As already indicated, with the advent of research governance, the identification of a sponsor for research is now mandatory. In the absence of an external funding body then an NHS trust or a university may take responsibility as a sponsor and this is especially the case where NHS employees are undertaking small-scale research studies as part of an educational programme.

Accountability to sponsors can be manifest through the establishment of research project steering groups and advisory groups. Generally speaking, advisory groups merely advise, whereas steering groups can actually dictate the direction of a project. While accountability in these cases, for funding purposes, is ultimately to the funder, there will be intermediate and very close accountability of the researcher to steering and advisory groups and meeting arrangements with these groups may be specified within a contract.

The contract should also specify the terms and conditions of the grant. The sponsor should make clear exactly what the grant is supporting (and what it is not), when accounts and reports are due, and in what form. In most cases, the usual expectation is for a final report to be submitted by a specified date but, in longer studies, interim reports might be required. A sponsor has every right to dictate the conditions of the grant. It is in the researcher's own interests to know exactly what is being expected and to accept the grant only if the sponsor's conditions are acceptable and manageable.

Particular care needs to be taken in this respect when research sponsorship is provided by a commercial organisation. The *Code of Professional Conduct* (NMC 2002b) warns nurses to:

> ensure that your registration is not used in the promotion of commercial products or services, (to) declare any financial or other interests in relevant organisations providing such goods or services and ensure that your professional judgement is not influenced by any commercial considerations.

Thus, for example, special care would be required to maintain a totally objective stance in a research project on infant feeding which was funded by a manufacturer of artificial milk products. Freedom to publish the results (irrespective of the findings) should be established as the researcher's right at the outset, in circumstances of this kind. In relation to this kind of issue, the guidelines provided by the Royal College of Nursing (1998b) advise that the 'researcher does not necessarily guarantee solutions to problems, and should make explicit the limitations and likely benefits of the proposed research'.

Once agreed, the sponsor's conditions are set out in a letter or, in the case of larger grant-giving bodies, in a formal contract. Before the grant is released this kind of document is usually required to be signed by all parties who will be held accountable by the sponsor for the satisfactory completion of the project and the agreed deployment of the funds. Failure to comply with the conditions of grant during the course of the project could result in withdrawal of the sponsor's support. If there is failure to complete the work satisfactorily, or to deliver the agreed 'products', it is likely that the researcher(s) concerned would be deemed ineligible to apply for funds from that grant-giving body for future research. Thus, a researcher's relationship with the sponsor, whether in a direct or indirect line of accountability, is a formal contractual relationship. As such, it should be clearly defined and understood from the outset.

Accountability to research ethics committees

There is a similarly formal process of accountability in relation to research ethics committees. Undertaking any nursing research project which involves human subjects or the use of NHS facilities requires the prior approval of the appropriate research ethics committee or committees. The role of these committees is to ensure that all research in the healthcare field is ethically sound. In order to obtain ethical approval, the researcher submits an application outlining the research protocol and detailing the ethical implications of the proposed study and the procedures that will be followed to ensure that the undertaking will be ethically sound. Currently ethics committees are organised into local research ethics committees (LRECs) and multicentre research ethics committees (MRECs) and the latter deal with applications which would otherwise have to be submitted to five or more LRECs. The arrangements at local and national levels for the conduct of ethics committees in the UK are currently under review and information can be obtained from the Central Office of Ethics Committees (COREC: www.corec.org.uk).

What is ethical research?
A short but helpful account of the ethical principles underpinning research is provided in the introduction to the booklet on ethics related to research in nursing (RCN, 1998b), which was formulated by the Research Advisory Group (now the Research Society) of the Royal College of Nursing. Beneficence (doing good to people) and non-maleficence (doing them no harm) are identified as two ethical principles of major importance in research. According to Thompson *et al.* (1994), 'in order to be ethical, nursing research must be based on prior assessment of risks and benefits of the research procedures' and they argue that a research project 'would not be justified when the risks outweigh the benefits'.

Assuming that the proposed research fulfils these fundamental conditions, other ethical principles of importance (as mentioned in the RCN booklet) include the principle of fidelity (trust), because research subjects entrust themselves to the researcher; the principle of autonomy (self-determination), which underpins the condition of voluntary informed consent; the principle of veracity (truth-telling), which is crucial in terms of the information given to patients as well as in the eventual reporting of the research; and, of course, the principle of confidentiality which, in research as in other spheres of professional practice, has legal as well as ethical dimensions.

Research can be designed from the outset to be ethically sound if steps are taken to address each of these principles in the course of developing a research proposal. There are, of course, some research topics and designs which have an inherently complex ethical dimension. Some client groups (for example, children, the mentally ill, frail older people and the dying) pose particularly difficult moral dilemmas for the researcher. These need to be resolved if the researcher is to be morally accountable, and indeed the concepts of ethics and accountability are inextricably linked.

Being 'morally accountable'
In a formal sense, the researcher's 'moral accountability' is to the research ethics committee. When the committee grants ethical approval there is the expectation that the researcher will conduct the research exactly as planned, including adhering to any procedures designed specifically to safeguard ethical soundness. Occasionally ethics committees do engage in direct monitoring of the conduct of the approved research; sometimes they require periodic progress reports; but more often the ethical conduct of the research is entrusted to the researcher. Thus, moral accountability depends essentially on the personal integrity of the individual researcher.

Even for the most conscientious individual this can be taxing. Take, for example, a project in which frail older people are involved and, because of their recognised vulnerability, the ethics committee has been particularly demanding about the procedure to be used for ensuring that informed voluntary consent is obtained. First, there is the task of deciding what information about the research must be given to the potential subjects, and how it should be presented. The information must be presented very clearly (whether verbally or in writing, or both) and it must be sufficient in detail but, for older people, not overly complicated, as this may cause confusion or unnecessary anxiety. Then there is the need to work out a practical procedure for imparting the information and obtaining the patient's consent, usually involving a formal signature.

In theory the procedure is simple enough, but in practice it can be less than straightforward. On initial approach, older patients may be wary of the whole idea of research or, in contrast, willing to submit unquestioningly to any request, especially one coming from a nurse. Should the former be subjected to persuasion and the latter encouraged to exercise caution? And what of the older person who is quite happy to sign the consent form but does not seem to have studied (or understood) the information? In any case, how does the researcher ever really know that the given consent is truly both informed and voluntary? Any researcher, quite naturally, feels under pressure to recruit the required number of subjects, and when the procedures which were approved by the ethics committee have been dutifully followed, there is every temptation to accept consent at face value and to set aside any niggling doubts about its authenticity.

Being morally accountable is a demanding aspect of research. Ethics committees have an important role to play in safeguarding the ethical soundness of research, but the maintenance of ethical standards is largely dependent on the discretion and integrity of the individual researcher. Even elaborate research governance arrangements will not overcome this and will not prevent rogue researchers from conducting unethical and even harmful research or research which has not been properly approved (Watson & Manthorpe, 2002).

Accountability to research participants

Grant-giving bodies and research ethics committees are in positions of authority and have a degree of 'hold' over the researcher's exercise of accountability. However, the subjects of research are in a relatively powerless position. Attention has been drawn already to the distinction between duty and dueness in accountability.

Acknowledgement of the dependence of research subjects is especially important in nursing and health services research. It is usually the case that research subjects are recruited while they are patients, whether in hospital or at home. As such they occupy a position of dependence in the system (as distinct from a position of authority or equality). Patients may thus feel a sense of obligation to participate in the research.

Basic principles

The nurse researcher, as nurse, will safeguard the interests of patients if guided by the essential principles of the NMC *Code of Professional Conduct* (2002b). The code states that as a registered nurse or midwife 'you must act to identify and minimise the risk to patients or clients'. Such a basic principle is as pertinent to the work of a nurse researcher as it is to that of any practising nurse.

The former UKCC *Code of Professional Conduct* for the registered nurse (UKCC, 1992a) also pointed out the necessity to 'avoid any abuse of your privileged relationship with patients and clients and of the privileged access allowed to their person, property, residence or workplace'. This is an important principle, particularly for nurses who are engaged in 'on-the-job' research and are recruiting for research purposes those patients with whom they are already involved as practitioners. In such situations, clear delineation, for the patient, of the nurse's dual roles is imperative if abuse of the nurse's pre-existing privileged relationship and access is to be avoided.

A nurse researcher 'from outside', of course, does not have such a relationship. In our experience, however, patients do tend to accord a nurse researcher the kind of sympathy and willingness to oblige that they tend to give nurses in general. There may be merit, therefore, in the researcher concealing their identity as a nurse, particularly if there is no reason in terms of the patient's interests why this should be declared. However, in the experience of one of the authors (RW) it is increasingly being demanded by ethics committees that the person approaching a patient directly about involvement in research, and even in data collection, is the nurse caring for the patient. This, of course, produces an immediate conflict of interest – even if this is just at the level of an initial approach or in seeking informed consent.

Respecting autonomy

In exercising accountability to research participants, respect for their autonomy is a basic premise. The necessity for, and importance of, involving research subjects on the basis of informed voluntary consent has already been emphasised. On this subject, the RCN (1998b) spells out what is involved:

> Researchers are responsible for obtaining freely given and informed consent from each individual who is to be a subject of study or, in some other way, personally involved in the research. This requires that the researcher explain as fully as possible, and in terms meaningful to the subjects, the nature and purpose of the study, how and why they were selected and invited to take part, what is required of them and who is undertaking and financing the investigation. This information should be provided in written form at all times; the subject's consent, whether written or verbal, should be recorded.

Further, the RCN guidelines draw attention to the fact that respect for the autonomy of research participants is an ongoing responsibility of the researcher:

In seeking voluntary informed consent, the researcher must emphasise that the subjects have an absolute right to refuse to participate or to withdraw from the study at any time without their care being affected in any way. The rights of refusal and withdrawal must be totally respected by researchers.

In exercising accountability in research, therefore, the matter of respect for the autonomy of participants is of paramount importance.

Fulfilling pledges of confidentiality

Another key issue that concerns accountability to research subjects is confidentiality. The NMC *Code of Professional Conduct* makes clear that, in the exercise of professional accountability, the nurse must 'protect confidential information'. The RCN research ethics guidelines (RCN, 1998b) draw attention to the fact that 'researchers should be aware that personal health information, such as medical records and nursing notes, is confidential and therefore permission and consent are required for its use in research'. Further, the guidelines point out that 'the nature of any promises of confidentiality or restriction on the use of data must be made clear to the subjects and subsequently strictly adhered to by the researcher'. Thus, the fulfilment of any pledge of confidentiality is an important dimension of accountability in research.

It is relatively easy to promise confidentiality of personal information which is collected in the course of a research project when subjects are part of a large sample and the data are quantitative in nature and, as such, reduced to collective numerical results. In such research – typically a survey – it is almost impossible for individual subjects to be identified in the final report. Nevertheless, this needs to be explained carefully to a potential subject who, unfamiliar with the process of data analysis, may not understand how personal information will be reduced to an anonymous form. Reassurance must also be given about how such data will be stored safely in the interim, for example, under a code number rather than by name. Such reassurance is particularly important if very personal or controversial data are being collected, or if the research participants are (or feel) especially vulnerable. This may be the case, for example, when a study is concerned with people who have HIV infection or AIDS, or when patients are being invited by a researcher to be openly critical of the care they have received, or when nursing students still on course are being asked to evaluate their education programme.

The confidentiality of data gathered for research is much more difficult to guarantee in the case of a small sample or a setting-specific study. When the sample is small, personal data are less easy to reduce to anonymity and, in a time-specific research report, an individual subject conceivably could be identified on the basis of even a limited number of straightforward details such as age, sex, occupation and medical diagnosis. Similarly, it can be difficult to conceal the identity of the location of a setting-specific study. It does not take too much detective work for a reader to track down a study location when, for example, it is described by an Edinburgh-based researcher as a 20-bedded male surgical ward in a large, local teaching hospital. Better, in our view, that pledges of confidentiality and anonymity are not given in such cases. It may well be that individual subjects and staff in particular settings will have no objection to being potentially identifiable in the research report. Whatever is decided, the researcher must be able to exercise accountability for the agreed procedures regarding the protection of confidential information which is collected for purposes of the research.

Being accountable when anonymity cannot be assured

Protecting the confidentiality of data collected in the course of a small-sample qualitative research study, however, is inherently difficult. It is possible that the researcher will be unable to guarantee anonymity, and this must be cleared in advance with the informants so that they consent to participation knowing that their accounts may be personally identifiable. In such cases, the researcher's accountability to the subjects is put to the most stringent of tests.

The personal dilemmas and discomfort that may be experienced by the researcher in such a situation were described by Bergum (1991) who undertook a phenomenological study of the real-life experiences of women in the transition through pregnancy, childbirth and early mothering. Her data derive from a series of conversations over time with six women. Bergum writes about the tension for a phenomenological researcher between the 'inner person' and the 'outer activities'. She reflects that:

> the ethical commitments to these women permeated my mind and my actions throughout the study and still continue. . . . Using their stories for my research purposes binds me to them in a way that goes beyond the technical considerations of how to handle the raw data of research.

Bergum also points out that in the published version of her study the women are not 'anonymous' to themselves and their words are 'available to (them) for continued reflection'. Thus, in a study such as this, private lives become public, and personal development is recorded for all time.

In qualitative studies it is sometimes the practice for the researcher to return the subjects' accounts to them for scrutiny. In doing so, the researcher is choosing to exercise accountability at a personal level to each of the participants in a way that does not occur in other forms of research. In principle, however, the same degree of personal accountability to subjects is present (theoretically, at least) in all research. The fact that research subjects generally do not have the opportunity to scrutinise and challenge the researcher's account and interpretation of the data does not lessen the researcher's responsibility to report the data truthfully, and thereby to fulfil their final responsibility in the process of accountability to the research participants.

On the other hand, the participation of users of health services in setting research agendas, approving projects and participating in steering groups is increasing and this is a central plank of current UK Government policy with regard to health research. The research governance framework (Department of Health, 2001f) also requires researchers to specify the extent of user involvement in their research.

Accountability to research 'gatekeepers'

Although potential participants in nursing and health services research are protected from exploitation by the requirement that a researcher obtains their personal consent to involvement, there is prior protection afforded by 'gatekeepers', through whom researchers must negotiate access before approaching potential subjects. This is necessary even when the proposed research has gained the approval of a funding body and of the relevant research ethics committee(s).

Who are the 'gatekeepers'

'Gatekeepers' control a researcher's access to potential subjects, to a site or to information. In nursing research access to all three is usually required. In the health service, both practitioners and managers can act as gatekeepers. Indeed, even the initial access to these personnel may have to be sought in the first instance from higher authority. In some regions, for example, it may be expected that that director of nursing at the health board level should be the first line of approach when a researcher wishes to discuss a proposed research project with managers in a chosen site in that area. In the case of research involving nursing students, the head of school may act as the gatekeeper. Having obtained their permission, the researcher then pursues access downwards through the hierarchy to the local site selected for undertaking the proposed research.

Negotiating access in this way can be a time-consuming process, but it does provide protection for patients and staff. Quite reasonably, a manager acting as a gatekeeper may rule that the entry of a researcher into a particular clinical area at a particular time and for a particular purpose without good reason, is not acceptable. Thus, a request for research access may be refused. One assumes that such a managerial decision will have taken due account of the views of the charge nurse and senior medical staff, and, indeed, that their views would carry most weight in the case of research to be conducted in their clinical area.

All requests for research access are now considered at NHS trust level by a research committee operating under research governance procedures (Department of Health, 2001f). There should be the expectation that all requests for access to conduct scientifically sound and justifiable research will be received sympathetically and assessed objectively. There is no justification for research access to be denied on the basis of a manager's whim or a charge nurse's general lack of interest in research.

Some of the influences that affect the decision making of gatekeepers were discussed by Mander (1992b) in the light of her own experiences in seeking access for a study of midwives' care of mothers whose babies were relinquished for adoption. Although she won the support of midwife managers with ease, some social workers were less cooperative. Like one of the research ethics committees involved, a hospital social worker failed to appreciate the relevance of the study to midwifery; and social workers in a local authority agency were not prepared to allow access to mothers contemplating relinquishment of their babies on grounds that the research would add further stress to an already very stressful situation. Mander advises that, when deciding whether or not to permit research access, the gatekeepers should recognise when their own experience is lacking or their views are based on mere assumptions. In such cases, she suggests, 'they should take advantage of the opportunity to draw on the expertise of those with different or more wide-ranging experience'. Mander's experience may be less likely to occur now, given that health professionals are more aware of research and research governance is more transparent

Changing relationships with 'gatekeepers'

The gatekeeping role within UK healthcare research has now been entirely placed within one framework, research governance, and this framework is operated within every NHS trust. The framework covers all aspects of research from some of those already mentioned, such as sponsorship and user involvement, but also covers the ethical aspects of the study, the management arrangements, the scientific scrutiny and the financial probity. Ethics committees remain independent of research governance, but the latter cannot operate without ethical committee approval. The UK Government has also published comprehensive governance arrangements for research ethics committees, intended to streamline and standardise the current system.

In the current climate of encouragement for more collaboration between researchers and service-based personnel in the NHS, it is theoretically possible that the process of negotiation for research access will become less, rather than more, difficult. As managers and practitioners become more aware of the importance attached to research in the health service, they are becoming more positive about facilitating it. It is likely, too, that the planning of research will more commonly become a joint enterprise. Thus, it will become less common for a researcher to finalise a research protocol and then begin the process of seeking access 'from cold'.

It is conceivable that trusts may become less willing to grant access for independent research which may produce findings that could disadvantage their position in the healthcare market. Trusts may choose, therefore, to rely increasingly on in-house research, or commissioned work over which internal control of results can be obtained. Another possibility is that a trust would continue to grant access to independent researchers but with conditions attached that limit the researcher's freedom to publish and, thereby, publicise the results. This experience has already been reported by one experienced nurse researcher who presented research results to her NHS employers – who had commissioned the research – but she had difficulty publishing these because the results were not favourable to her employers (Robinson, 2002).

The researcher's accountability to 'gatekeepers'
In the same way as a researcher has ongoing and specific accountability to their sponsor and to the research ethics committee, there is continuing accountability to the research gatekeepers even after access has been granted. Access will have been granted on the basis of an agreed plan of investigation. The researcher is therefore bound to work within that agreed plan and, in exercising accountability, should not extend beyond the boundaries of that agreement and must adhere closely to the agreed procedures (for example, the procedure for obtaining informed voluntary consent).

Very often, for reasons beyond the control of the researcher, the research plan has to be modified in the course of the project. For example, the sampling procedure that was piloted may not be working because the patient population in the study setting has changed as a consequence of a new admissions policy within the hospital. Or, perhaps, the method of non-participant observation which had been developed for use in the practice nurse's clinic in a health centre is proving to be too intrusive, even although it had been acceptable to staff and patients when piloted. In other cases, it might be that the promised cooperation of staff (for example, to randomise a nursing intervention) is impossible to maintain because of new pressures or the introduction of new working methods within the ward. In such cases the researcher has the choice of abandoning the project or changing strategy. Either way, the decision must be made in consultation with the gatekeepers (and then with the approval of the sponsor and the ethics committees) if the researcher's accountability to those in positions of authority is to be maintained. Under the research governance framework researchers will be asked for periodic reports on the number of subjects they have recruited into studies and also on any changes to the protocol of the study.

On completion of the work, the researcher should provide the gatekeepers with an account of the research findings. This may have to await the approval of the sponsor and it may require a modified form of reporting in order to preserve promised confidentiality to patients or staff, who may be recognised by insiders even although they are impossible to identify from the outside. On this point, the RCN's (1998b) ethical guidelines for nursing research emphasise that: 'any promises of anonymity or confidentiality given to the participants by the researcher must be respected also by the nurse commissioning or agreeing to a study being carried out'. The guidelines continue: 'No attempt should be made to probe data or results in order to identify any individual, instance or place which has been concealed deliberately by the researcher.' Nurses in positions of authority where research is carried out are also advised that 'deviations from expected uncovered in the course of research should not be used by managers for punitive purposes although remedial actions would be expected to follow'. Thus, by this analysis, the researcher's accountability to the research participants takes priority.

Accountability to (and of) the profession

Like nurses in any sphere of professional practice, nurse researchers can be considered to be accountable to their peers. It would have to be said that nurse researchers have not been held in particularly high esteem by the profession. They have been criticised for being 'ivory-towered' and out of touch with the real world of nursing. The topics of their research have been described as irrelevant and there has been much criticism of their perceived inability to communicate their findings in ways that are meaningful to practising nurses. For their part, researchers have retaliated by criticising the profession's lack of interest in research. This mutual lack of understanding was very much in evidence in the 1980s and even into the 1990s.

Changing relationships

More recently there has been an evident improvement in the relationship between the doers and the consumers of research. There is no doubt that nurse researchers have become very aware of the need for their research to have (and be seen to have) direct relevance to practice and service delivery issues, and for the findings to be reported in ways that nursing colleagues find interesting and meaningful to their everyday work.

For their part, practising nurses have become more appreciative of the contribution and limitations of research as, gradually, education at basic and post-basic levels has improved the extent of research awareness and knowledge throughout the profession. Research has now become a component of job descriptions in nursing and, as a result, practising nurses and nurses in management have come to appreciate that nurse researchers have expertise which is otherwise in short supply in the profession.

The development of this mutual appreciation is welcome. Some successful initiatives in collaborative working have been reported. It is just these sorts of interactive relationships that were encouraged in the Research and Development Strategy for the NHS.

Towards shared accountability for research

As the gap between research and practice continues to close it can be expected that the profession will come to see itself as sharing accountability for nursing research with its researchers. In the past it may have been reasonable for nurse researchers to be blamed for the lack of impact of research, or its lack of relevance, but this is no longer an appropriate stance for the profession to adopt.

It was argued at the beginning of the chapter that any accountable profession must assume responsibility for the ongoing development of its knowledge base. It follows, therefore, that it is the profession's responsibility to ensure that its infrastructure supports research; that it possesses an adequate research capability; and that the research undertaken is relevant, and is disseminated and utilised effectively.

The formulation of the *Strategy for Research in Nursing, Midwifery and Health Visiting* (discussed earlier) was evidence that the profession has taken on this responsibility. Built into the strategy, the task force spelt out the respective responsibilities for research of managers, teachers, practitioners and researchers. Also, in 1993, nursing's professional organisation in the United Kingdom, the RCN, established a research committee with the purpose of strengthening and coordinating the RCN's contribution to, and support of, research in nursing.

These were important landmarks in the profession's development in terms of its commitment to research. Thus, in the 1990s, accountability for research was seen, for the first time, as a collective responsibility of the profession as a whole and not just its researchers. And, in recent years, this movement has continued steadily, with a comprehensive research and development strategy for nursing and midwifery now being in place (or under formulation) in each of the four countries of the UK.

Accountability to the wider public

Since awareness of the importance of research in nursing is relatively new, it is not surprising that it does not yet feature largely in the public image of nursing. Most lay people still perceive nursing as being an essentially practical occupation, more in need of kind hearts than clever heads. This view seems to be common even among people in similarly practical fields of work, such as engineering, computing, accountancy and dentistry, in which the role of research is taken for granted.

It is no wonder, really, that lay people have such a poor appreciation of the nature and relevance of nursing research. Rarely has there been any mass media coverage in this country of the results of a nursing research study. One of the authors (AJT) was pleased but startled when she read a magazine report of a piece of research she had done concerning the experiences and information needs of women who were undergoing chemotherapy for breast cancer (Tierney *et al.*, 1989). Why should she have been startled? In almost every daily newspaper there are reports of medical and scientific research. Every year, there is detailed news coverage of the proceedings of the British Psychological Society's scientific meeting. Why has nursing research not been similarly reported in the public domain? This is something that should be remedied if we want to improve public recognition of the role of research in nursing and, indeed, of the whole changing nature of nursing practice and nursing education.

The nursing profession has long enjoyed the support of the British public and, in the current era of health service reform, the continuation of that support is vital. The place and importance of research in nursing needs to be explained. Many members of the public may be unaware that nursing services are the largest single item of health service expenditure. If there was a greater awareness of this fact, it is likely that the public would appreciate the crucial role that research can (and needs to) play in demonstrating the worth and value of nursing. Indeed, the public may be quicker than the profession itself has been to appreciate that such research is, a priori, a responsibility of a publicly accountable profession.

Tensions of multiple accountability

Accountability in research has been examined in relation to a number of different parties: the sponsor, research ethics committees, research participants, gatekeepers, the profession and the wider public. Some of these parties are in positions of authority (for example, the sponsor and the gatekeepers), whereas others are in positions of dependence (i.e. participating patients). Depending on their positions, the researcher's accountability derives from duty or dueness and, correspondingly, it is more or less regulated by formal mechanisms or ethical conventions. When an individual is required to exercise different types of accountability to a number of parties – as, in terms of this analysis, is the case for a nurse researcher – there are, inevitably, inherent tensions.

The tensions of multiple accountability in nursing research are probably felt most acutely by nurses who are engaged in on-the-job research. In such a situation the key tensions arise from the individual's dual role as nurse *and* researcher. In relation to clinical responsibilities, the nurse is accountable to the employing organisation through the usual channels. In relation to parallel research responsibilities, there may be formal accountability to an external sponsor or supervisor. Conflicts of interest may arise.

The RCN research ethics guidelines (1998b) offer useful advice for nurses in such a position. They state:

> When research is undertaken in the context of an organisational structure, it is important to clarify in advance the responsibilities of the researcher within the organisation, the lines of communication and the means of settling any conflicts of interest which may arise.

Conflicts of interest do arise. How does the nurse fulfil accountability to meet the completion deadline set by the research sponsor when the pressing demands of clinical work eat into the time that has been agreed for the research? Can the nurse always fulfil accountability to the research subjects in terms of confidentiality of data when that same data may be recognised as being potentially crucial to the patient's medical or nursing care? What does the nurse do when research uncovers colleagues acting unethically or negligently? And when a patient, as research subject, breaks down in distress is it possible to maintain the detached stance expected of a researcher, or should the nurse offer the type of professional counsel which would be appropriate to the role of practitioner?

The role of a nurse researcher who is not also carrying clinical responsibilities is, in contrast, less complicated. On this, the RCN guidelines state that 'the nurse who is undertaking a research project in an exclusively research role has no responsibility for the service, care, treatment or advice given to patients or clients unless stipulated within the design of the research'. In theory this is perfectly correct, and a nurse researcher would not be held accountable for patient care. The guidelines make clear that 'any intervention in a professional capacity should be confined to situations in which a patient or client requires to be protected or rescued from danger'.

In practice, however, it can be difficult to decide what constitutes 'danger'. Reasonably, a nurse researcher may feel that it is better to err on the safe side and to act as a nurse rather than be criticised later for foolishly maintaining a 'stand-off' position as a researcher. After all, the NMC (2002b) *Code of Professional Conduct* states that: 'in caring for patients and clients, you must act to identify and minimise risk to patients and clients.' Could a researcher who is also a nurse ever be expected to act at odds with this?

In a hospital ward, or other environment in which the research subjects are patients under care, it is usually easy for the nurse researcher, without breaching confidentiality, to find a way of conveying any anxieties to staff or encouraging patients themselves to pass on information that the researcher feels, in the patient's interest, should be known to staff. In one study which one of us supervised (AJT), the research assistant who was interviewing older patients in a hospital ward kept meeting patients who, when asked, reported that they were suffering from pain, sometimes to a considerable degree. Sticking closely to her instructions to behave as a researcher, she had not conveyed her concern to staff. It was not in the interests of the research to alert staff to the apparent need for better pain management because the aim of the study was to obtain baseline data prior to the introduction of potential improvements. As nurses, however, we did not feel we could continue to collect evidence of inadequate pain control without alerting the ward staff, and so this was done.

Much more difficult dilemmas arose in the course of a study which involved interviews at home with older patients who had been recently discharged from hospital (Tierney *et al.*, 1993). An experienced health visitor was employed to undertake these interviews and it was emphasised that her role was as a researcher. Contingency plans were agreed in case, in her professional judgement, she considered any of the subjects to be in difficulty and in need of care or attention. The main strategy was that she would advise the older person (or the carer) to contact the GP. If they were unwilling to do so, she would ask their permission to contact the GP herself. A number of the older people were found to be in dire straits, and the contingency plans proved to be satisfactory in most cases.

There were instances, however, when the researcher did not consider there was a real danger but, as a health visitor, she felt compelled to offer professional advice and, occasionally, to give hands-on care. There were also circumstances which had not been anticipated. For example, there were occasions when there was no answer when the researcher arrived at the prearranged time to undertake the interview. Did she just go away and bemoan the loss of an interview and the waste of time? No: as a health visitor with a keenly developed sense of professional accountability she did whatever was necessary to ensure that the older person was safely elsewhere or, if in the house, was not in danger or in need of help.

These examples are not especially dramatic. They do illustrate, however, that there are tensions for the nurse researcher – irrespective of which is the primary role – between accountability as a researcher and accountability as a nurse.

Conclusion

Nursing research continues to grow in volume and prestige. Research training or appreciation is integral to most nursing curricula, but research capacity remains low. The early years of this century have seen genuine efforts by the Departments of Health and the Higher Education funding bodies to redress the low research capacity and it is probably safe to assume that the volume and the quality of nursing research will continue to grow. Increasing research activity will bring more nurses into contact with research governance procedures and research committees. This will raise awareness across the profession, of the elements of accountability – scientific, ethical and financial – which involvement in nursing research necessarily carries.

Appendix

Nursing & Midwifery Council Code of professional conduct

Protecting the public through professional standards

Code of professional conduct

As a registered nurse, midwife or health visitor, you are personally accountable for your practice. In caring for patients and clients, you must:

- respect the patient or client as an individual
- obtain consent before you give any treatment or care
- protect confidential information
- cooperate with others in the team
- maintain your professional knowledge and competence
- be trustworthy
- act to identify and minimise risk to patients and clients

These are the shared values of all the United Kingdom healthcare regulatory bodies.

This *Code of professional conduct* was published by the Nursing and Midwifery Council in April 2002 and came into effect on 1 June 2002.

Introduction

1.1 The purpose of the *Code of professional conduct* is to:

- inform the professions of the standard of professional conduct required of them in the exercise of their professional accountability and practice
- inform the public, other professions and employers of the standard of professional conduct that they can expect of a registered practitioner.

1.2 As a registered nurse, midwife or health visitor, you must:

- protect and support the health of individual patients and clients
- protect and support the health of the wider community

- act in such a way that justifies the trust and confidence the public have in you
- uphold and enhance the good reputation of the professions

1.3 You are personally accountable for your practice. This means that you are answerable for your actions and omissions, regardless of advice or directions from another professional.
1.4 You have a duty of care to your patients and clients, who are entitled to receive safe and competent care.
1.5 You must adhere to the laws of the country in which you are practising.

2 As a registered nurse, midwife or health visitor, you must respect the patient or client as an individual

2.1 You must recognise and respect the role of patients and clients as partners in their care and the contribution they can make to it. This involves identifying their preferences regarding care and respecting these within the limits of professional practice, existing legislation, resources and the goals of the therapeutic relationship.
2.2 You are personally accountable for ensuring that you promote and protect the interests and dignity of patients and clients, irrespective of gender, age, race, ability, sexuality, economic status, lifestyle, culture and religious or political beliefs.
2.3 You must, at all times, maintain appropriate professional boundaries in the relationships you have with patients and clients. You must ensure that all aspects of the relationship focus exclusively upon the needs of the patient or client.
2.4 You must promote the interests of patients and clients. This includes helping individuals and groups gain access to health and social care, information and support relevant to their needs.
2.5 You must report to a relevant person or authority, at the earliest possible time, any conscientious objection that may be relevant to your professional practice. You must continue to provide care to the best of your ability until alternative arrangements are implemented.

3 As a registered nurse, midwife or health visitor, you must obtain consent before you give any treatment or care

3.1 All patients and clients have a right to receive information about their condition. You must be sensitive to their needs and respect the wishes of those who refuse or are unable to receive information about their condition. Information should be accurate, truthful and presented in such a way as to make it easily understood. You may need to seek legal or professional advice, or guidance from your employer, in relation to the giving or withholding of consent.
3.2 You must respect patients' and clients' autonomy – their right to decide whether or not to undergo any healthcare intervention – even

where a refusal may result in harm or death to themselves or a foetus, unless a court of law orders to the contrary. This right is protected in law, although in circumstances where the health of the foetus would be severely compromised by any refusal to give consent, it would be appropriate to discuss this matter fully within the team, and possibly to seek external advice and guidance (see clause 4).

3.3 When obtaining valid consent, you must be sure that it is:

- given by a legally competent person
- given voluntarily
- informed

3.4 You should presume that every patient and client is legally competent unless otherwise assessed by a suitably qualified practitioner. A patient or client who is legally competent can understand and retain treatment information and can use it to make an informed choice.

3.5 Those who are legally competent may give consent in writing, orally or by cooperation. They may also refuse consent. You must ensure that all your discussions and associated decisions relating to obtaining consent are documented in the patient's or client's healthcare records.

3.6 When patients or clients are no longer legally competent and thus have lost the capacity to consent to or refuse treatment and care, you should try to find out whether they have previously indicated preferences in an advance statement. You must respect any refusal of treatment or care given when they were legally competent, provided that the decision is clearly applicable to the present circumstances and that there is no reason to believe that they have changed their minds. When such a statement is not available, the patients' or clients' wishes, if known, should be taken into account. If these wishes are not known, the criteria for treatment must be that it is in their best interests.

3.7 The principles of obtaining consent apply equally to those people who have a mental illness. Whilst you should be involved in their assessment, it will also be necessary to involve relevant people close to them; this may include a psychiatrist. When patients and clients are detained under statutory powers (mental health acts), you must ensure that you know the circumstances and safeguards needed for providing treatment and care without consent.

3.8 In emergencies where treatment is necessary to preserve life, you may provide care without patients' or clients' consent, if they are unable to give it, provided you can demonstrate that you are acting in their best interests.

3.9 No one has the right to give consent on behalf of another competent adult. In relation to obtaining consent for a child, the involvement of those with parental responsibility in the consent procedure is usually necessary, but will depend on the age and understanding of the child. If the child is under the age of 16 in England and Wales, 12 in Scotland and 17 in Northern Ireland, you must be aware of legislation and local protocols relating to consent.

3.10 Usually the individual performing a procedure should be the person to obtain the patient's or client's consent. In certain circumstances, you may seek consent on behalf of colleagues if you have been specially trained for that specific area of practice.

3.11 You must ensure that the use of complementary or alternative therapies is safe and in the interests of patients and clients. This must be discussed with the team as part of the therapeutic process and the patient or client must consent to their use.

4 As a registered nurse, midwife or health visitor, you must cooperate with others in the team

4.1 The team includes the patient or client, the patient's or client's family, informal carers and health and social care professionals in the National Health Service, independent and voluntary sectors.

4.2 You are expected to work cooperatively within teams and to respect the skills, expertise and contributions of your colleagues. You must treat them fairly and without discrimination.

4.3 You must communicate effectively and share your knowledge, skill and expertise with other members of the team as required for the benefit of patients and clients.

4.4 Healthcare records are a tool of communication within the team. You must ensure that the healthcare record for the patient or client is an accurate account of treatment, care planning and delivery. It should be consecutive, written with the involvement of the patient or client wherever practicable and completed as soon as possible after an event has occurred. It should provide clear evidence of the care planned, the decisions made, the care delivered and the information shared.

4.5 When working as a member of a team, you remain accountable for your professional conduct, any care you provide and any omission on your part.

4.6 You may be expected to delegate care delivery to others who are not registered nurses or midwives. Such delegation must not compromise existing care but must be directed to meeting the needs and serving the interests of patients and clients. You remain accountable for the appropriateness of the delegation, for ensuring that the person who does the work is able to do it and that adequate supervision or support is provided.

4.7 You have a duty to cooperate with internal and external investigations.

5 As a registered nurse, midwife or health visitor, you must protect confidential information

5.1 You must treat information about patients and clients as confidential and use it only for the purposes for which it was given. As it is impractical to obtain consent every time you need to share information with others, you should ensure that patients and clients understand that some information may be made available to other members of the team involved in the delivery of care. You must guard against breaches of confidentiality by protecting information from improper disclosure at all times.

5.2 You should seek patients' and clients' wishes regarding the sharing of information with their family and others. When a patient or client is considered incapable of giving permission, you should consult relevant colleagues.

5.3 If you are required to disclose information outside the team that will have personal consequences for patients or clients, you must obtain their consent. If the patient or client withholds consent, or if consent cannot be obtained for whatever reason, disclosures may be made only where:

- they can be justified in the public interest (usually where disclosure is essential to protect the patient or client or someone else from the risk of significant harm)
- they are required by law or by order of a court.

5.4 Where there is an issue of child protection, you must act at all times in accordance with national and local policies.

6 As a registered nurse, midwife or health visitor, you must maintain your professional knowledge and competence

6.1 You must keep your knowledge and skills up to date throughout your working life. In particular, you should take part regularly in learning activities that develop your competence and performance.

6.2 To practise competently, you must possess the knowledge, skills and abilities required for lawful, safe and effective practice without direct supervision. You must acknowledge the limits of your professional competence and only undertake practice and accept responsibilities for those activities in which you are competent.

6.3 If an aspect of practice is beyond your level of competence or outside your area of registration, you must obtain help and supervision from a competent practitioner until you and your employer consider that you have acquired the requisite knowledge and skill.

6.4 You have a duty to facilitate students of nursing and midwifery and others to develop their competence.

6.5 You have a responsibility to deliver care based on current evidence, best practice and, where applicable, validated research when it is available.

7 **As a registered nurse, midwife or health visitor, you must be trustworthy**

    7.1 You must behave in a way that upholds the reputation of the professions. Behaviour that compromises this reputation may call your registration into question even if it is not directly connected to your professional practice.

    7.2 You must ensure that your registration status is not used in the promotion of commercial products or services, declare any financial or other interests in relevant organisations providing such goods or services and ensure that your professional judgement is not influenced by any commercial considerations.

    7.3 When providing advice regarding any product or service relating to your professional role or area of practice, you must be aware of the risk that, on account of your professional title or qualification, you could be perceived by the patient or client as endorsing the product. You should fully explain the advantages and disadvantages of alternative products so that the patient or client can make an informed choice. Where you recommend a specific product, you must ensure that your advice is based on evidence and is not for your own commercial gain.

    7.4 You must refuse any gift, favour or hospitality that might be interpreted, now or in the future, as an attempt to obtain preferential consideration.

    7.5 You must neither ask for nor accept loans from patients, clients or their relatives and friends.

8 **As a registered nurse, midwife or health visitor, you must act to identify and minimise the risk to patients and clients**

    8.1 You must work with other members of the team to promote health-care environments that are conducive to safe, therapeutic and ethical practice.

    8.2 You must act quickly to protect patients and clients from risk if you have good reason to believe that you or a colleague, from your own or another profession, may not be fit to practise for reasons of conduct, health or competence. You should be aware of the terms of legislation that offer protection for people who raise concerns about health and safety issues.

    8.3 Where you cannot remedy circumstances in the environment of care that could jeopardise standards of practice, you must report them to a senior person with sufficient authority to manage them and also, in the case of midwifery, to the supervisor of midwives. This must be supported by a written record.

    8.4 When working as a manager, you have a duty toward patients and clients, colleagues, the wider community and the organisation in which you and your colleagues work. When facing professional dilemmas, your first consideration in all activities must be the interests and safety of patients and clients.

8.5 In an emergency, in or outside the work setting, you have a professional duty to provide care. The care provided would be judged against what could reasonably be expected from someone with your knowledge, skills and abilities when placed in those particular circumstances.

Glossary

Accountable	Responsible for something or to someone.
Care	To provide help or comfort.
Competent	Possessing the skills and abilities required for lawful, safe and effective professional practice without direct supervision.
Patient and client	Any individual or group using a health service.
Reasonable	The case of *Bolam v. Friern Hospital Management Committee* (1957) produced the following definition of what is reasonable. 'The test is the standard of the ordinary skilled man exercising and professing to have that special skill. A man need not possess the highest expert skill at the risk of being found negligent . . . it is sufficient if he exercises the skill of an ordinary man exercising that particular art.' This definition is supported and clarified by the case of *Bolitho v. City and Hackney Health Authority* (1997).

Further information

This *Code of professional conduct* is available on the Nursing and Midwifery Council's website at: www.nmc-uk.org. Printed copies can be obtained by writing to the Publications Department, Nursing and Midwifery Council, 23 Portland Place, London W1B 1PZ, by fax on 020 7436 2924 or by email at: publications@nmc-uk.org. A wide range of NMC standards and guidance publications expand upon and develop many of the professional issues and themes identified in the *Code of professional conduct*. All are available on the NMC's website. A list of current NMC publications is available either on the website or on request from the Publications Department as above.

Enquiries about the issues addressed in the *Code of professional conduct* should be directed in the first instance to the NMC's professional advice service at the address above, by email at: advice@nmc-uk.org, by telephone on 020 7333 6541/6550/6553 or by fax on 020 7333 6538.

The Nursing and Midwifery Council will keep this *Code of professional conduct* under review and any comments, suggestions or requests for further clarification are welcome, both from practitioners and members of the public. These should be addressed to the Director of Policy and Standards, NMC, 23 Portland Place, London W1B 1PZ.

April 2002

Summary

As a registered nurse, midwife or health visitor, you must:

- respect the patient or client as an individual
- obtain consent before you give any treatment or care
- cooperate with others in the team
- protect confidential information
- maintain your professional knowledge and competence
- be trustworthy
- act to identify and minimise the risk to patients and clients

References

Abbott, A. (1988) *The System of Professions: An essay on the division of expert labour.* University of Chicago Press, Chicago.

Abel-Smith, B. (1960) *A History of the Nursing Profession.* Heinemann, London.

Acheson, D. (1998) *Independent inquiry into inequalities in health report.* The Stationery Office, London.

Adams, C. & Forester, S. (2002) *Clinical governance in primary care and public health practice.* Community Practitioners and Health Visitor's Association, London.

Alaszewski, A. (2000) Risk in nursing practice: developing and sustaining trust. In: *Managing Risk in Community Practice: Nursing, Risk and Decision Making* (eds Alaszewski, A., Alasewski, H., Ayer, S. & Manthorpe, J.) Bailliere Tindall, London.

Alaszewski, A., Gates, B., Motherby, E., Manthorpe, J. & Ayer, S. (2001) *Educational preparation for learning disability nursing: Outcome Evaluation of the Contribution of Learning Disability Nurses within the Multi-Professional, Multi-Agency Team.* ENB Research Highlights, English National Board for Nursing, Midwifery and Health Visiting, London.

Alaszewski, A., Alaszewski, H., Manthorpe, J. & Ayer, S. (1997) *Assessing and Managing Risk in Nursing Education and Practice: Supporting Vulnerable People in the Community.* ENB Research Highlights, English National Board for Nursing, Midwifery and Health Visiting, London.

Alberti, K. (2001) 'Medical errors: a common problem'. *British Medical Journal,* **322,** March, 501–2.

Alderson, P. (1990) *Choosing for Children.* Oxford University Press, Oxford.

Alderson, P. (1993) *Children's Consent to Surgery.* Open University Press, Milton Keynes.

Alderson, P. (1996) *Healthcare choices: making decisions with children.* Institute for Public Policy Research, London.

Alderson, P. (2000) *Young children's rights: exploring beliefs, principles and practice.* Jessica Kingsley, London.

Allen, P. (2000) Accountability for clinical governance: developing collective responsibility for quality in primary care. *British Medical Journal,* **321,** 608–11.

Altschul, A. (1972) *Patient-Nurse Interaction.* Churchill Livingstone, Edinburgh.

Altschul, A. (1999) Editorial. *Journal of Psychiatric and Mental Health Nursing,* **6** (4), 261–3.

Amnesty International (1995) *Childhood Stolen – grave human rights violations against children.* Amnesty International British Section, London.

Angell, V. (1990) 'Prisoners of technology: the case of Nancy Cruzan, New England'. *Journal of Medicine*, **332**, 1226–8.

Anthony, R. & Govindarajan, V. (1998) *Management Control Systems*, 9th edn. Irwin McGraw Hill.

Anthony, W.A. (1993) 'Recovery from mental illness: the guiding vision of the mental health service system in the 1990s'. *Psychosocial Rehabilitation Journal*, **16** (4), 11–23.

Appleby, F. & Sayer, L. (2001) Public health nursing – health visiting. In: *Community health care nursing* (eds Sines, D., Appleby, F. & Raymond, E.), 2nd edn. Blackwell Science, London.

Archard, D. (1993) *Children: Rights and Childhood*. Routledge, London.

Aristotle, (1962) *Nicomachean Ethics*. Bobbs-Merrill Educational Publishing Ltd, Indianapolis.

Atherton, H. (2002) A History of Learning Disability, Chapter 3. In: *Learning Disabilities* (ed. Gates, B.), 4th edn. Churchill Livingstone, Edinburgh.

Ballinger, C. & Payne, S. (2002) 'The construction of the risk of falling among and by older people'. *Ageing and Society*, **22**, 305–24.

Baly, M. (1986) *Florence Nightingale and the Nursing Legacy*. Croom Helm, London.

Barker, P. (1989) 'Reflections on the philosophy of caring in mental health'. *International Journal of Nursing Studies*, **26** (2), 131–41.

Barker, P. (2001) 'The Tidal Model: developing an empowering person-centred approach to recovery within psychiatric and mental health nursing'. *Journal of Psychiatric and Mental Health Nursing*, **8** (3), 233–40.

Barker, P.J. & Reynolds, B. (1996) 'Rediscovering the proper focus of nursing – a critique of Gournay's position on nursing theory and models'. *Journal of Psychiatric and Mental Health Nursing*, **3** (1), 76–80.

Barker, P. (2002) 'Doing what needs to be done. A respectful response to Burnard and Grant'. *Journal of Psychiatric and Mental Health Nursing*, **9** (2), 232–6.

Bartlett, W. & Le Grand, J. (1993) 'The Performance of Trusts'. In: *Evaluating the NHS Reforms* (eds Robinson, R. & Le Grand, J.). Kings Fund Institute, London.

Batey, M. & Lewis, F. (1982) 'Clarifying autonomy and accountability in nursing service', part 1. *Journal of Nursing Administration*, **12** (9), 13–18.

Beech, B.A.L. & Thomas, P. (1999) 'The witch hunt: an international persecution of quality midwifery'. *AIMS Journal* **11** (2), 1, 3–4.

Benson, E.R. (1990) Nineteenth Century Women, the Neophyte Nursing Profession, and the World's Columbian Exposition of 1893. In: *Florence Nightingale and her Era* (eds Bullough, V., Bullough, B. & Stanton, M.P.), pp. 108–22. Garland, New York.

Bergman, R. (1981) 'Accountability: definitions and dimensions'. *International Nursing Review*, **28**, 53–8.

Bergum, V. (1991) Being a phenomenological researcher. In: *Qualitative Nursing Research* (ed. Morse, J.M.), pp. 5–71. Sage, London.

Bernauer, J. (1987) Michel Foucalt's ecstatic thinking. In: *The Final Foucalt* (eds Bernauer, J. & Rasmussen, D.). The MIT Press, Cambridge, Massachusetts.

Bines, W. & Lightfoot, J. (1999) School nursing – an evaluation of policy and practice. In: *Evaluating community nursing* (eds Atkin, K., Lunt, N. & Thompson C.). Bailliere Tindall, London.

Bogle, I. (2002) http://www.dailytelegraph.co.uk/news/main.jhtml?xml=/news/2002/10/17/nhs17.xml&sSheet=/news/2002/10/17/ixnewstop.html

Bolam Test (1957) *Bolam v. Friern HMC (1957)*, 2 All England Reports 118.

Botes, S. (1998) 'The CPHVA view of health visiting and the new NHS'. *Community Practitioner*, **71** (6), 220–2.

BJN (1903) 'The International Council of Nurses'. *The British Journal of Nursing*, 21 Nov., 409.

BJN (1915a) 'The National Council of Trained Nurses of Great Britain and Ireland and the care of the sick and wounded. Resolution and statement sent to the Secretary of State for War'. *The British Journal of Nursing*, 30 Jan., Supplement, i–vii.

BJN (1915b) 'The State needs Nurses'. *The British Journal of Nursing*, 27 March, 245.

BMJ (2000) 'Reducing error, improving safety'. *British Medical Journal*, **321**, August, 505–8.

Bristol Royal Infirmary Inquiry (2001) *Learning from Bristol: The report of the public inquiry into children's heart surgery at the Bristol Royal Infirmary, 1984–1995*. Cm 5207. The Stationery Office, London.

Brocklehurst, N. & Walshe, K. (1999) Quality and the new NHS. *Nursing Standard*, **13** (51), 46–51.

Brownlee, M., Mackintosh, C.L., Wallace, E.M., Johnstone, F.D., Murphy-Black, T. (1996) 'A survey of interprofessional communication in a labour suite'. *British Journal of Midwifery*, **4**, 492–5.

Brykczyñska, G. (2000) 'Not quite the judgement of Solomon'. *Paediatric Nursing*, **12** (9), 6–8.

Burden, B. & Jones, T. (2001) 'Improvements to supervision are essential for best practice'. *British Journal of Midwifery*, **9**, 220–6.

Buttigieg, M. (1997) 'Advanced nursing in a primary care led NHS'. *Health Visitor*, **70**, 68–70.

Cabell, C. (1992) 'The efficacy of primary nursing as a foundation for patient advocacy'. *Nursing Practice*, **5** (3), 2–5.

Campbell, P. (2000) The consumer of mental health care. In: *Mental Health Nursing: an evidence-based approach* (eds Newall, R. & Gournay, K.), pp. 11–26. Churchill Livingstone, Edinburgh.

Carpenter, D. (1992) 'Advocacy'. *Nursing Times*, **88** (27), 1–8.

Carter, G.B. (1939) *A New Deal for Nurses*. Gollancz, London.

Casey, A. (1993) Development and use of the partnership model of nursing care. In: *Advances in Child Health Nursing* (eds Glasper, A. & Tucker, A.), pp. 183–9. Scutari Press, Harrow.

CDO (2002) Cambridge International Dictionary of English. Cambridge Dictionaries, Online http://dictionary.cambridge.org/ (Accessed 8 March 2002).

CETHV (1977) *An investigation into the principles of health visiting*. Council for the Education and Training of Health Visitors, London.

Champion, R. (1991) 'Educational Accountability – What ho the 1990s!' *Nurse Education Today*, **11**, 407–14.

Chapple, A., Rogers, A., MacDonald, W. & Sergison, M. (2000) Patient's perceptions of changing professional boundaries and the future of 'nurse-led' services. *Primary Health Care Research and Development*, **1**, 39–50.

Christensen, P.J. & Kenney, J.W. (1995) *Nursing Process: Application of Conceptual Models*. Mosby, St Louis.

Clark, J. (2000) *Accountability in Nursing*, Second WHO Ministerial Conference on Nursing and Midwifery in Europe, Munich, 15–17 June 2000.

Clarke, A., Woodhouse, K. & Millar, B. (2001) 'Best of British'. *Community Practitioner*, 74, 246–50.

Clarridge, A., Boran, S. & Bninski, M. (2001) Contemporary issues in district nursing. In: *Community health care nursing* (eds Sines, D., Appleby, F. & Raymond, E.), 2nd edn. Blackwell Science, London.

Clinical Standards Board for Scotland (2001) *Clinical Standards for Schizophrenia.* CSBS, Edinburgh.

Clinical Standards Board for Scotland (2002) *Frequently asked questions*: http://www.clinicalstandards.org/faq.html

Closs, S.J. & Cheater, F. M. (1999) 'Evidence for nursing practice: a clarification of the issues'. *Journal of Advanced Nursing*, 30, 10–17.

Clothier, C. (1994) *The Allitt Inquiry – Independent inquiry relating to deaths and injuries on the children's ward at Grantham and Kesteven General Hospital during the period February to April 1991.* HMSO, London.

Cochrane, A.L. (with Blythe M.) (1989) 'One Man's Medicine'. *British Medical Journal*, London (Memoir Club), p. 82. Cited on: http://www.cochrane.de/cochrane/archieco.htm

Cole, A. & Oxtoby, K. (2002) 'Patient Power'. *Nursing Times*, 98 (51), 22–5.

Commission for Health Improvement (2001) *A Guide to Clinical Governance Reviews.* Commission for Health Improvement, London.

Commission for Health Improvement (2002) *Review codes and assessment scale.* Commission for Health Improvement, London.

Community Practitioners' and Health Visitors' Association (2001) *A suvey of community nurses access to internet and email.* Community Practitioners' and Health Visitors' Association, London.

Cook, E.T. (1913) *The Life of Florence Nightingale.* vol. 2. MacMillan, London.

Cook, P. (1990) 'Who's accountable?' *Journal of District Nursing*, June, 18–20.

Cooper, J. & Harpin, V. (1991) *This is our child.* Oxford University Press, Oxford.

Cowley, S. (1993) 'Skill mix: value for whom?' *Health visitor*, 66, 166–8.

Cowley, S. & Andrews, A. (2001) 'A scenario-based analysis of health visiting dilemmas'. *Community Practitioner*, 74, 139–42.

Crofts, L. & McMahon, A. (2000) *Raising the profile of nursing research amongst medical research charities.* Royal College of Nursing, London.

Cummins, R.A. (1997) 'Self-rated Quality of Life Scales for People with Intellectual Disability: A Review. *Journal of Applied Research in Intellectual Disabilities*, 10, 199–216.

Davies, H. & Mannion, R. (2000) Clinical Governance: Striking a Balance between Checking and Trusting. In: *Reforming Markets in Healthcare: An Economic Perspective* (ed. Smith, P.). Open University Press, Buckingham.

Dawson, P.J. (1997) 'A reply to Kevin Gournay's "Schizophrenia: a review of the contemporary literature and implications for mental health nursing theory, practice and education"'. *Journal of Psychiatric and Mental Health Nursing*, 4 (1), 1–8.

Day, P. & Klein, R. (1987) *Accountabilities: Five Public Services.* Tavistock, London.

de la Cuesta, C. (1994) 'Relationships in health visiting: enabling and mediating'. *International Journal of Nursing Studies*, 31 (5), 451–9.

Department of Health (1989) *Working for Patients.* Department of Health, London.

Department of Health (1990) *General Practice in the National Health Service: a new contract.* HMSO, London.

Department of Health (1991) *Research for Health.* HMSO, London.

Department of Health (1992) *The Health of the Nation.* HMSO, London.

Department of Health (1993a) *The Challenges for Nursing and Midwifery in the Twenty-first Century.* HMSO, London.

Department of Health (1993b) *Report of the Task Force on the Strategy for Research in Nursing, Midwifery and Health Visiting.* Department of Health, Research and Development Division, London.

Department of Health (1993c) *Changing Childbirth. Report of the expert maternity group.* Department of Health, London.

Department of Health (1994a) *Corporate Governance in the NHS: Code of Conduct – Code of Accountability.* Department of Health, London.

Department of Health (1994b) *Negotiating school health services.* The Stationery Office, London.

Department of Health (1996) *Clinical Negligence Costs* (FDL(96)39). NHSE, London.

Department of Health (1997) *The New NHS: Modern, Dependable.* Cm 3807, HMSO, London.

Department of Health (1998) *A First Class Service: Quality in the New NHS.* HMSO, London.

Department of Health Scotland (1998) *Working together for a healthier Scotland.* The Stationery Office, Edinburgh.

Department of Health Wales (1998) *Better health, better Wales.* The Stationery Office, Cardiff.

Department of Health (1999a) *Clinical Governance: quality in the new NHS.* Department of the Health, London.

Department of Health (1999b) *For the Record: Managing records in the NHS Trusts and Health Authorities.* HSC 1999/053. NHSE, London.

Department of Health (1999c) *Saving lives: our healthier nation.* Cmnd.4386. The Stationery Office, London.

Department of Health (1999d) *Review of the prescribing, supply and administration of medicines.* Chair Dr. J. Crown. The Stationery Office, London.

Department of Health (1999e) *Making a Difference: Strengthening the nursing, midwifery and health visiting contribution to health and healthcare.* The Stationary Office, London.

Department of Health (2000a) *Research and development for a first class service.* Department of Health, London.

Department of Health (2000b) *The NHS Plan: A Plan for Investment – A Plan for Reform.* The Stationery Office, London.

Department of Health (2000c) *An Organisation with a Memory: Report of an expert group on learning from adverse events in the NHS.* The Stationery Office, London.

Department of Health (2001a) *Clinical Negligence: What are the Issues and Options for Reform?* Department of Health, London: http://www.doh.gov.uk/clinicalnegligencereform/index.htm

Department of Health (2001b) *National service framework for older people.* The Stationery Office, London.

Department of Health (2001c) *Valuing People: A New Strategy for Learning Disability for the Twenty-first Century.* Cm. 5086. HMSO, London.

Department of Health (2001d) *Seeking Consent: Working with People with Learning Disabilities*. HMSO, London.

Department of Health (2001e) *Research Governance Implementation Plan*. HMSO, London.

Department of Health (2001f) *Research Governance Framework for Health and Social Care*. Department of Health, London.

Department of Health (2001g) *Health Service Circular/2001/00*. Department of Health, November 2002.

Department of Health (2002a) *The NHS Plan*. The Stationery Office, London.

Department of Health (2002b) *Liberating the talents. Helping primary care trusts and nurses to deliver the NHS plan*. Department of Health, London.

Department of Health (2003) *Making Amends: A Consultation Paper Setting out Proposals for Reforming the Approach to Clinical Negligence Litigation*. A report by the Chief Medical Officer, June, Department of Health, London.

Department of Health SSPS (2000) *Investing for health. A consultation document*. DHSSPS, Edinburgh.

Dickerson, M. (1997) The reality of clinical supervision. In: *Contemporary Community Nursing* (eds Burley, S., Mitchell, E.E., Melling, M., Smith, M. Chilton, S. & Crumplin, C.). Arnold, London.

Dingwall, R., Rafferty, A.M. & Webster, C. (1988) *An Introduction to the Social History of Nursing*. Routledge, London.

Dock, L.L. (1899) 'Nursing in England'. *The Nursing Record and Hospital World*, 11 November, 395–7.

Dock, L.L. (1901) *American Journal of Nursing*, 865.

Dock L.L. (1912) *A History of Nursing*. Vol. 3. Putnam, New York.

Donaldson, L.J. & Muir Gray, J.A. (1998) 'Clinical Governance: a quality duty for health organisations'. *Quality in Healthcare*, 7 (suppl), S37–44.

Donnison, J. (1988) *Midwives and medical men: a history of the struggle for the control of childbirth*. New Barnet Historical Publications, London.

Duerden, J. (2002) Supervision at the beginning of a new century, Chapter 5. In: *Failure to Progress: The contraction of the midwifery profession* (eds Mander, R. & Fleming, V.). Routledge, London.

Dyer, C. (1985) 'The Gillick Judgment, contraception and the under 16s: House of Lords Ruling'. *British Medical Journal*, **291**, 1208–9.

Eaton, L. (2002) 'NICE accused of restricting treatment for eye patients'. *British Medical Journal*, **325**, 853.

Elcoat, C. & Raymond, B. (2001) 'Does clinical governance make any difference to patient care?' *Nursing Times*, **97** (16), 15.

Ellis, R. & Whittington, D. (1993) *Quality Assurance in Health Care: a handbook*. Edward Arnold, London.

Emmanuel, C., Otley, D. & Merchant, K. (1990) *Accounting for Management Control*, 2nd edn. Chapman Hall, London.

Etuk, E. (2001) 'Professionalism and accountability'. *The Practising Midwife*, **4** (7), 28–30.

Etzioni, A. (1975) Epilogue: alternative conceptions of accountability. In: *Accountability in Health Facilities* (ed. Greenfield, H.I.), pp. 121–42. Praeger, New York.

Evans, A. (1993) 'Accountability: a core concept for primary nursing'. *Journal of Advanced Nursing*, **2**, 231–4.

Fasting, U., Christensen, J. & Glending, S. (1998) 'Children sold for Transplants: Medical and Legal Aspects'. *Nursing Ethics*, 5, 518–26.

Fenwick, Mrs Bedford (1887) Address to hospital matrons 10 December (reprinted). *British Journal of Nursing*, 15 May 1920, p. 288.

Fenwick, Mrs Bedford (1897) 'The better organisation of the nursing profession'. *Nursing Record and Hospital World*, 6 November, 369–71 and 13 November, 389–91.

Fenwick, Mrs Bedford (1901a) 'A plea for the higher education of trained nurses'. *Transactions of the Third International Congress of Nurses Pan-American Exposition*. Buffalo, New York State, USA, 18–21 September, pp. 363–9.

Fenwick, Mrs Bedford (1901b) 'The organisation and registration of nurses'. *Transactions of the Third International Congress of Nurses Pan-American Exposition*, Buffalo, 18–21 September, pp. 339–40.

Ferlie, E., Pettigrew, A. & Ashburner, L. (1996) *The New Public Management in Action*. Oxford University Press, Oxford.

Florin, D. & Rosen, R. (1999) 'Evaluating NHS Direct'. *British Medical Journal*, 19, 5–6.

Forester, S. (2002) *Delegation and Professional Accountability*. Professional Briefing, London Community Practitioners' and Health Visitors' Association.

Foucault, M. (1979) *Discipline and Punish*. Peregrine, Harmondsworth.

Foucault, M. (1980) 'About the beginning of the hermeneutics of the self'. Lecture delivered at Dartmouth College, New Hampshire, USA, 17 & 24 November 1980. Transcript T. Keenan & M. Blasius. In: Carrette, J. (1999) *Religion and culture by Michel Foucault*. Manchester University Press, Manchester.

Foucault, M. (1985) *The use of pleasure: the history of sexuality*. Vol. 2. Pantheon, New York.

Foucalt, M. (1988) Technologies of the self. In: *Technologies of the self: a seminar with Michel Foucalt* (eds Martin, L., Gutman, H. & Hutton, P.). The University of Massachusetts Press, Amhurst.

French, P. (1993) *Responsibility Matters*. Kansas University Press, Lawrence.

Gallant, M., Beaulieu, M. & Carnevale, F. (2002) 'Partnership: an analysis of the concept with the nurse–client relationship'. *Journal of Advanced Nursing*, 40, 149–57.

Gardner, L. (1998) 'Leading primary care: time for action'. *Health Visitor*, 71, 21–2.

Garwood Gowers, A. Lewis, T. & Tingle, J. (2001) *Healthcare Law: The Impact of the Human Rights Act 1998*. Cavendish Publishing, London.

Gates, B. (1994) *Advocacy: A Nurses' Guide*. Scutari Press, London.

Gates, B. (1997) Understanding Learning Disability. In: *Learning Disabilities* (ed. Gates, B.), 3rd edn. Churchill Livingstone, Edinburgh.

Gates, B. (2001) Advocacy. In: *Mental Health Nursing: An evidence based approach* (eds Newell, R. & Gournay, K.), pp. 373–89. Churchill Livingstone, Edinburgh.

General Medical Council (2001) *Good Medical Practice*, 3rd edn. GMC, London. http://www.gmc-uk.org/standards/good.htm

Glasper, A. & Tucker, A. (eds) (1993) *Advances in Child Health Nursing*. Scutari Press, Harrow.

Glover, D. (1999) 'Accountability'. *Nursing Times Monographs* No. 27. NT Books, London.

Glover, J. (1970) *Responsibility*. Routledge & Kegan Paul, London.

Goer, H. (1995) *Obstetric myths versus research realities.* Bergin & Garvey, Westport.

Goldberg, D. (2000) Foreword. In: *Mental Health Nursing: An evidence based approach* (eds Newell, R. & Gournay, K.). Churchill Livingstone, Edinburgh.

Goodman, N.W. (1998) 'Sacred Cows: To the abattoir – clinical governance'. *British Medical Journal*, **317**, 1725.

Gournay, K. (1995) 'What to do with nursing models'. *Journal of Psychiatric and Mental Health Nursing*, **2** (5), 325–7.

Gournay, K. (1996) 'Schizophrenia: a review of contemporary literature and implications for mental health nursing theory, practice and education'. *Journal of Psychiatric and Mental Health Nursing*, **3** (1), 7–12.

Gournay, K. (1997) 'Responses to "what to do with nursing models – a reply from Gournay"'. *Journal of Psychiatric and Mental Health Nursing*, **4** (3), 227–31.

Gournay, K. (2003) 'Review of Evidence in Mental Health Care by Priebe, S. and Slade, M.' *Journal of Psychiatric and Mental Health Nursing*, **10**, 247–9.

Gray, J.A.M. (2001) *Evidence Based Healthcare*, 2nd edn. Churchill Livingstone, Edinburgh.

Gray, J.D. & Donaldson, L. (1996) 'Improving the Quality of Healthcare through Contracting: a study of health authority practice'. *Quality in Healthcare*, **5**, 201–5.

Greenfield, H.I. (1975) *Accountability in Health Facilities.* Praeger, New York.

Griffiths, R. (1983) *NHS Management Enquiry.* Department of Health and Social Security, London.

Haines, A. & Jones, R. (1994) 'Implementing Findings of Research'. *British Medical Journal*, **308**, 488–92.

Haldane, E. (1923) *The British Nurse in Peace and War.* Murray, London.

Hall, J. (1999) 'Home birth: the midwife effect'. *British Journal of Midwifery*, **7**, 4225–7.

Halligan, A. & Donaldson, L. (2001) 'Implementing clinical governance: turning vision into reality'. *British Medical Journal*, **322**, 1413–17.

Hanley, J. (2002) Analysis of questionnaires on capacity for nursing and midwifery research in HEIs and NHS Trusts. Personal Communication.

Helmstadter, C. (1993) 'Old nurses and new: nursing in the London teaching hospitals before and after the mid-nineteenth-century reforms'. *Nursing History Review*, **1**, 43–70.

Her Majesty's Government (1989) *The Children Act.* HMSO, London.

Her Majesty's Government (1991) *Convention on the Rights of the Child.* Adopted by the General Assembly of the United Nations 20 November 1989. HMSO, London.

Higher Education Funding Council for England (2001) *Research in nursing and allied health professions.* Higher Education Funding Council for England, London.

HM Government (1991) Convention on the Rights of the child adopted by the General Assembly of the United Nations, 20 November 1989. HMSO, London.

HMSO (1972) *Report of the Committee on Nursing* (The Briggs Report). HMSO, London.

Hobby, C. (2001) *Whistleblowing and the Public Interest Disclosure Act 1998.* Institute of Employment Rights, London.

Home Office (1998) *Supporting Families.* The Stationery Office, London.

Hood, C. (1995) 'The new Public Management in the 1980s: variations on a theme'. *Accounting, Organisations and Society*, **20** (2/3), 93–109.

Hopton, J. & Heaney, D. (1999) 'Towards primary care groups. The development of local healthcare cooperatives in Scotland'. *British Medical Journal*, **318**, 1185–7.

Hopwood, A. (1984) Accounting and the pursuit of efficiency. In: *Issues in Public Sector Accounting* (eds Hopweed, A. & Tompkins, C.). Philip Alan, Oxford.

Hoskin, K. & Macve, R. (1986) 'Accounting and the Examination: a genealogy of disciplinary power'. *Accounting, organisations and society*, **12**, 105–36.

House of Commons (1992) *Health Committee Second Report, Maternity Services*, (Winterton Report). HMSO, London.

Humphrey, C., Miller, P. & Scapens, R. (1993) 'Accountability and accountable management in the UK Public Sector'. *Accounting, Auditing and Accountability Journal*, **6** (3), 7–29.

Hunt, G. (1997) 'The human condition of the professional: discretion and accountability'. *Nursing Ethics*, **4** (6), 519–26.

Hunt, G. (1998) *Whistleblowing in the social services: public accountability and professional practice*. Edward Arnold, London.

Hunter, B. (1998) 'Professional issues. Independent midwifery – future inspiration or relic of the past?' *British Journal of Midwifery*, **6**, 85–7.

Hutchinson, S.A. (1989) 'Responsible Subversion: a study of rule bending among nurses'. *Scholarly Inquiry for Nursing Practice*, **4** (1), 3–17.

Isherwood, K. (1988) 'Friend or watchdog?' *Nursing Times*, **84** (24), 65.

Isherwood, K. (1989) 'Independent midwifery in the UK'. *Midwife, Health Visitor and Community Nurse*, **25**, 307–9.

Jacobs, K. & Walker, S. (2000) Accounting and Accountability in the Iona Community, *Sixth Interdisciplinary Perspectives on Accounting Conference*, Manchester, 9–12 July 2000.

James, A. & Prout, A. (1990) *Constructing and Reconstructing Childhood: Contemporary Issues in the Sociological Study of Childhood*. Falmer Press, London.

James, J.W. (1979) Isabel Hampton and the professionalisation of nursing in the 1980s. In: *The Therapeutic Revolution* (eds Rosenburg, C.R. & Vogel, M.J.), pp. 201–44. University of Pennsylvania Press, Philadelphia.

Jones, M.A. (2002) *Textbook on Torts*, 8th edn. Oxford University Press, Oxford.

Jones, S.R. (1994) *Ethics in Midwifery*. Mosby, London.

Kelson, M. (1997) *User Involvement: a practical guide to developing effective user involvement strategies in the NHS College of Health*. The Research Unit of the Royal College of Physicians, London.

Kendall, S.(1999) Evidence-based health visiting – the utilisation of research for effective practice. In: *Research issues in community nursing* (ed. McIntosh, J.). Macmillan, London.

Kent, A., Gates, B. & Thompson, J. (2002) *Final Report of the Learning Disability Education and Training Project*. The East Yorkshire Learning Disability Institute, The University of Hull, Hull.

Kitzinger, J.V., Green, J.M. & Coupland, V.A. (1990) Labour relations: midwives and doctors on the labour ward. In: *The Politics of Maternity Care: Services for Childbearing Women in the Twentieth Century* (eds Garcia, J., Kilpatrick, R. & Richards, M.), pp. 149–62. Oxford University Press, Oxford.

Klein, R. & Redmayne, S. (1992) *Patterns of Priorities: a Study of the Purchasing and Rationing Policies of Health Authorities*. National Association of Health Authorities and Trusts (NAHAT) Research Paper No 7, NAHAT, Birmingham.

Klein, R. (2001) *The New Politics of the NHS*. Person Education, Essex.

Kmietowicz, Z. (2002) 'NICE widens patient group for leukemia drug'. *British Medical Journal*, **325**, 852.

Kohner, N. (1994) *Clinical supervision in practice*. King's Fund Centre, London.

Kubsch, S.M. (1996) 'Conflict, enactment, empowerment: conditions of independent therapeutic nursing intervention'. *Journal of Advanced Nursing*, **23**, 192–200.

Lanara, V. (1982) Responsibility in nursing. *International Nursing Review*, **29**, 7–10.

Lattimer, V., Sassi, F., George, S., Turnbull, J., Mullee, M. & Smith, H. (2000) 'Cost analysis of nurse telephone consultation in out of hours primary care: evidence from a randomised controlled trial'. *British Medical Journal*, **320**, 1053–7.

Lee, R. (1995) Resources and professional accountability. In: *Nursing Law and Ethics* (eds Tingle, J.H. & Cribb, A.), pp. 130–148. Blackwell Science, Oxford.

Lewis, F. & Batey, M.V. (1982) 'Clarifying autonomy and accountability in nursing services', Part 2. *Journal of Nursing Administration*, **12** (10), 10–15.

Lilley, R. (1999) *Making sense of clinical governance*. Radcliffe Medical Press, Oxford.

Littlejohns, P. (2001) The relationship between NICE and the national research and development programme. In: *Research and development for the NHS* (eds Baker, M.R. & Kirk, S.), pp. 39–58. Radcliffe Medical Press, Oxford.

Lloyd, G.E. (1969) *Aristotle: the Growth and Structure of His Thought*. Cambridge University Press, Cambridge.

Lockett, T. (1997) *Evidence-based and cost-effective medicine*. Radcliffe Medical Press, Oxford.

Loughlin, M. (2000) Quality and Excellence: meaning versus rhetoric. Chapter One. In: *Law and Medical Ethics* (eds Mason, J.K. & McCall-Smith, R.A.), 4th edn. Butterworths, London.

Luckes, E.C. (1914) *General Nursing*. Routledge & Kegan Paul, London.

Lugon, M. & Secker-Walker, J. (2001) *Advancing Clinical Governance*. The Royal Society of Medicine Press Limited, London.

Luker, K., Austin, L., Hogg, C., Ferguson, B. & Smith, K. (1997) 'Patients' views of nurse prescribing'. *Nursing Times*, **93** (17), 51–4.

Mason, J.K. & McCall-Smith, R.A. (1994) *Law and Medical Ethics*, 4th edn. Butterworths, London.

Mason, C. (2001) The public health agenda – can it really be part of community nursing? In: *Community nursing and healthcare. Insights and innovations* (ed. Hyde, V.). Arnold, London.

Mander, R. (1992a) 'See how they learn: experience as the basis of practice'. *Nurse Education Today*, **12**, 11–18.

Mander, R. (1992b) 'Seeking approval for research access: the gatekeeper's role in facilitating a study of the care of the relinquishing mother'. *Journal of Advanced Nursing*, **17**, 1460–4.

Mander, R. (1993) 'Autonomy in midwifery and maternity care'. *Midwives Chronicle*, **106** (1269), 369–74.

Manigan, P. (1993) 'Survival of the Fittest'. *Nursing Times*, **89** (6), 26.

McGann, S. (1992) *The Battle of the Nurses*. Scutari Press, London.

McIntosh, J., Lugton, J., Moriarty, D. & Carney, O. (1999) Exploring district nursing skills through research. In: *Research issues in community nursing* (ed. McIntosh, J.). Macmillan, London.

McLymont, M., Thomas, S. & Denham, M. (1986) *Health visiting and the elderly.* Churchill Livingstone, Edinburgh.

McSherry, R. & Haddock, J. (1999) 'Evidence-based health care: its place within clinical governance'. *British Journal of Nursing,* 8 (2), 113–17.

McSherry, R. & Pearce, P. (2002) *Clinical Governance.* Blackwell, Oxford.

Mead, G.H. (1934) *Mind Self and Society.* University of Chicago Press, Chicago.

Melia, C. (1995) Accountability – the ethical dimension. In: *Accountability in Nursing Practice* (ed. Watson, R.). Chapman and Hall, London.

Mental Health Commission (1998) *Blueprint for Mental Health Services in New Zealand – how things need to be done.* MHC, New Zealand.

Mental Health Commission (2002) Kia Mauri Tou! – Narratives of recovery from disabling mental health problems by Hilary Lapsley, Linda Waimarie Nikora and Rosanne Black: www.mhc.govt.nz/mhc

Merleau-Ponty, M. (1962) *The Phenomenology of Perception.* Routledge & Kegan Paul, London.

Miles, K. (1990) 'Health Authority Liable for Negligent Organisation of Maternity Services – *Bull v. Devon Health Authority,* Action for Victims of Medical Accidents'. *Medical Legal Journal,* **11**, 11.

Miller, J.A. (2001) Clinical governance. *Nursing Times Clinical Monographs,* No. 56. Macmillan, London.

Millerson, G. (1964) *The Qualifying Association.* Routledge, London.

Mishler, E. (1984) *The discourse of medicine: dialectics of medical interviews.* Ablex, Norwood.

Mollett, Miss (1898) (Matron of the Royal South Hants Infirmary) 'The duty of the matron to her profession'. *Nursing Record and Hospital World,* 25 June, 514.

Moore, D. (2001) 'Friend or Foe: A selective review of the literature concerning abuse of adults with learning disability by those employed to care for them'. *Journal of Learning Disabilities,* 5, 245–58.

Morten, H. (1895) *How to Become a Nurse.* Scientific Press, London.

Muir Gray, J.A. (1997) *Evidence Based Health Care: How to Make Health Policy and Management Decisions.* Churchill Livingstone, Edinburgh.

Mulligan, J. (1998) Attitudes towards the NHS and its alternatives, 1983–1996. In: *Healthcare UK 1997/98* (ed. Harrison, A.). Kings Fund, London.

Munro, R. & Mouritson, J. (1996) *Accountability: Power, ethos and the technologies of managing.* Thompson Business Press, London.

National Audit Office (2001) *Handling Clinical Negligence Claims in England.* HC 403, Session 2000–2001. The Stationery Office, London.

National Health Service Executive (1996a) *Promoting Clinical Effectiveness: a framework for action in and through the NHS.* The Stationary Office, London.

Newell, R. & Gournay, K. (2000) *Mental health nursing: An evidence-based approach.* Churchill Livingstone, Edinburgh.

Newson, K. (1986) 'Straight rules'. *Nursing Times,* **82** (27), 62–4.

NHS Management Executive Value for Money Unit (1993) *The Nursing Skill Mix in the District Nursing Service.* HMSO, London.

NHS Centre for Reviews and Dissemination (1996) *Undertaking Systematic Reviews of Research on Effectiveness.* CRD Report 4. NHS Centre for Reviews and Dissemination, University of York, York.

National Health Service Executive (1996b) *Risk Management in the NHS.* Department of Health, London.

NHS Centre for Reviews and Dissemination (1999) *Getting Evidence into Practice*, 5,1. NHS Centre for Reviews and Dissemination, University of York, York.

NHS Executive (1999a) *Making a difference: a strategy for nursing, midwifery and health visiting*. The Stationery Office, London.

National Health Service Executive (1999b) *Governance in the new NHS: Controls Assurance Statements 1999/2000*. HSC1999/123. Department of Health, London.

National Health Service Executive (2000) *Modernising Regulation: the New Nursing and Midwifery Council – a consultation document*. Department of Health, London.

Nursing & Midwifery Council (2002a) 'Indemnity Insurance: a matter of trust or a compulsory requirement?' *NMC News* Number 2. NMC, London.

Nursing & Midwifery Council (2002b) *The Code of Professional Conduct*. Nursing & Midwifery Council, London. http://www.nmc-uk.org/cms/content/publications/

Nursing Times (1921) 'Registration in other countries'. 19 March, 313.

Nuttall, J. (1993) *Punishment and Responsibility*. Polity Press, Cambridge.

OED (2002) Online English Dictionary: http://www.dictionary.com/ (Accessed 8 March 2002)

Office for Standards in Education (2002) Introduction to OFSTED: http://www.ofsted.gov.uk/about/intro.html

O'Neill, O. (2002) www.bbc.co.uk/radio4/reith2002/lecture3_text.shtml

Osbourne, D. & Gaebler, T. (1992) *Reinventing government: How the entrepreneurial spirit is transforming the public sector*. Plume Books, Penguin Group, New York.

Ouchi, W. (1979) 'A conceptual framework for the design of organisational control mechanisms'. *Management Science*, **25**, 833–48.

Parker, S. & Wilson, C. (1992) *An Introduction to Medicolegal Aspects of Practice Nursing*. Medical Defence Union, London.

Passos, J. (1973) 'Accountability: myth or mandate?' *Journal of Nursing Administration*, **3**, 17–22.

Pettinari, C.J. & Jessopp, L. (2001) ' "Your ears become your eyes": managing the absence of visibility in NHS direct'. *Journal of Advanced Nursing*, **36**, 668–75.

Picton, C. & Granby, T. (2002) Maintaining and developing competencies in nurse prescribing. *British Journal of Community Nursing*, **7**, 90–3.

Pollitt, C. & Bouckaert, G. (2000) *Public Management Reform: a comparative analysis*. Oxford University Press, Oxford.

Pollock, L. & Turner, G. (1998) *National depot neuroleptic audit project*. CRAG, Scottish Office, Edinburgh.

Power, M. (2000) The Evolution of the Audit Society, its politics of control & the advent of CHI. Chapter 9. In: *NICE, CHI & the NHS Reforms: Enabling Excellence or Imposing Control?* (eds Miles, A., Hampton, J.R. & Hurwitz, B.). Aesculapius Medical Press, London.

Prentice, S. (1994) 'Accountability in the NHS'. *Kings Fund News*, **17** (2), 2–3. Kings Fund, London.

Pritchard, A. & Kendrick, D. (2001) 'Practice nurse and health visitor management of acute minor illness in a general practice'. *Journal of Advanced Nursing*, **36**, 556–62.

Pyper, R. (1996) *Aspects of Accountability in the British System of Government*. Tudor Business Publishing, Eastham.

Repper, J. (2000) 'Adjusting the focus of mental health nursing: Incorporating service users' expeiences of recovery'. *Journal of Mental Health*, **9**, 575–87.

Reveley, S., Walsh, M. & Crumbie, A. (2002) 'Setting up a nurse practitioner service'. *Nursing Standard*, **17** (10), 33–7.

Robb, I.H. (1909) 'An international education standard for nurses'. *British Journal of Nursing*, 18 September, 233.

Roberts, J. (1991) 'The Possibilities of Accountability'. *Accounting, Organisations and Society*, **16**, 355–68.

Roberts, J. (1996) From discipline to dialogue: individualising and socialising forms of accountability. In: *Accountability: Power, ethos and the technologies of managing* (eds Munro, R. & Mouritson, J.). Thompson Business Press, London.

Robinson, J. (2002) Research for whom? In: *Exemplary research for nursing and midwifery* (eds Rafferty, A.M. & Traynor, M.), pp. 352–71. Routledge London.

Robinson, J., Watson, R. & Webb, C. (2002) 'The United Kingdom Research Assessment Exercise'. *Journal of Advanced Nursing*, **37**, 497–8.

Robinson, S., Golden, J. & Bradley, S. (1983) 'A Study of the Role and Responsibilities of the Midwife'. *Nursing Education Research Unit Report No. 1*, University of London, King's College, London.

Robinson, S. (1990) Maintaining the independence of the midwifery profession: a continuing struggle. In: *The Politics of Maternity Care: Services for Childbearing Women in the Twentieth Century* (eds Garcia, J., Kilpatrick, R. & Richards, M.), pp. 61–91. Clarendon Press, Oxford.

Rolfe, G. (1996) 'What to do with psychiatric nursing'. *Journal of Psychiatric and Mental Health Nursing*, **3** (5), 331–3.

Rothwell, H. (1996) 'Changing childbirth . . . changing nothing'. *Midwives* **109** (1306), 291–4.

Royal College of Nursing/Department of Health (1994) *Good practice in the administration of depot neuroleptics. A guidance document for mental health and practice nurses*. Health Publications Unit, RCN/DOH, Lancaster.

Royal College of Nursing (1998a) *Guidance for Nurses on Clinical Governance*. RCN, London.

Royal College of Nursing (1998b) *Ethics Related to Research in Nursing*. Scutari Press, London.

Royal College of Nursing (2000) *Clinical Governance: how nurses can get involved*. RCN, London.

Russell, B. (1991) *The Problems of Philosophy*. Oxford University Press, Oxford.

Ryan, D. (1985) The professional and the personal: Are they incompatible? In: *Accountable autonomy: Perspectives in professional education* (ed. Goodlad, S.), pp. 56–75. SRHE Annual Conference 1984. Society for Research into Higher Education, Guildford.

Ryan, D. (1993) 'Ambiguity in Nursing'. Seminar given to Department of Nursing Studies, University of Edinburgh, Edinburgh.

Ryan, D. (1997) Ambiguity in Nursing: The person and the organisation as contrasting sources of meaning in nursing. In: *The Mental Health Nurse: Views of Practice and Education* (ed. Tilley, S.), pp. 118–36. Blackwell Science, Oxford.

Ryan, D., Tilley, S. & Pollock, L. (1998) *Review of literature on the effectiveness of Community Psychiatric Nurses in achieving health outcomes for people with mental illness*. Department of Nursing Studies, The University of Edinburgh, Edinburgh.

Ryan, D. & Mowat, H. (2003) Introducing Scotland. *Spirited Scotland Newsletter,* 2, p. 3. http://www.spiritedscotland.org

Sackett, D.L., Richardson, W.S., Rosenberg, W. & Haynes, R.B. (1997) *Evidence based medicine.* Churchill Livingstone, New York.

Sang, B. & O'Neill, S. (2001) 'Patient involvement in clinical governance'. *British Journal of Health Care Management,* 7, 278–81.

Sargent, L. (2002) Practice and Autonomy, Chapter 3. In: *Failure to progress: the contraction of the midwifery profession* (eds Mander, R. & Fleming, V.). Routledge, London.

Saunders, M. (2001) General practice nursing. In: *Community health care nursing* (eds Sines, D., Appleby, F. & Raymond, E.), 2nd ed. Blackwell Science, London.

Scottish Executive Department of Health (1998) *Clinical Governance Arrangements.* NHS MEL (1998) 75, p. 2, Scottish Office, Edinburgh.

Scottish Executive Health Department (1998) *Designed to care – renewing the National Health Service in Scotland.* HMSO, Edinburgh.

Scottish Executive Health Department (2000a) *Our national health: a plan for action, a plan for change.* The Stationery Office, Edinburgh.

Scottish Executive Health Department (2000b) *Community care: a joint future.* The Stationery Office, Edinburgh.

Scottish Executive Health Department (2000c) *Clinical Governance.* MEL (2000) 29. The Stationery Office, Edinburgh.

Scottish Executive Health Department (2001a) *New Directions: Report on the Review of the Mental Health (Scotland) Act 1984.* HMSO, Edinburgh.

Scottish Executive Health Department (2001b) *Nursing for health: a review of the contribution of nurses, midwives and health visitors to improving the public's health in Scotland.* The Stationery Office, Edinburgh.

Scottish Executive Health Department (2001c) *Clinical Governance Arrangements.* NHS HDL (2001) 74. SEHD, Edinburgh.

Scottish Executive Health Department (2001d) *New Governance Arrangements in NHS in Scotland.* A Working Paper. SEHD, Edinburgh.

Scottish Executive Health Department (2002) *Nursing and Midwifery Research and Development Strategy.* The Stationery Office, Edinburgh.

Scottish Office Health Department (1997) *Framework for Mental Health Services in Scotland.* HMSO, Edinburgh.

Secretary of State for Health (2001) *Learning from Bristol – The Report of the Public Inquiry into children's heart surgery at the Bristol Royal Infirmary 1984–1995.* HMSO, London.

Sewall, M.W. (1905) 'How to lift your business into a profession' (address to the Matrons' Council in London 1899: reprinted). *American Journal of Nursing,* 6, 85–6.

Shaum, C., Humphreys, A., Wheeler, D., Cochrane, M., Skoda, S. & Clement, S. (2000) 'Nurse management of patients with minor illness in general practice: multicentre, randomised controlled trial'. *British Medical Journal,* 320, 1038–43.

Shipman Inquiry Reports (2002–2003) *Second Report, The Police Investigation of March 1998.* Cm 5853. The Stationery Office, London. For other reports see: http://www.the-shipman-inquiry.org.uk/reports.asp

Shotter, J. (1984) *Social Accountability and Selfhood.* Basil Blackwell, Oxford.

Sinclair, A. (1995) 'The Chameleon of Accountability: forms and discourses'. *Accounting, Organisations and Society,* 20, 219–37.

Sines, D. (2001) The context of community healthcare nursing. In: *Community health-care nursing* (eds Sines, D., Appleby, F. & Raymond, E.), 2nd edn. Blackwell Science, London.

Smith, J.P. (1981) Issues in nursing administration. In: *Current Issues in Nursing* (ed. Hockley, L.), pp. 64–78. Churchill Livingstone, Edinburgh.

Smith, S. (1998) 'Model Behaviour'. *Nursing management*, 5 (6), 19–24.

Spurgeon, P. (1997) 'How nurses can influence policy'. *Nursing Times*, 93 (45), 34–5.

Starkey, K. & McKinlay, A. (1998) Afterword: deconstructing organisation – discipline and desire. In: *Foucalt, management and organisation theory* (eds McKinlay, A. & Starkey, K.). Sage, London.

Stauch, M., Wheat, K. with Tingle, J. (2002) *Sourcebook on Medical Law*, 2nd edn. Cavendish Publishing, London.

Stewart, J. (1984) The Role of Information in Public Accountability. In: *Issues in Public Sector Accounting* (eds Hopwood, A. & Tomkins, C.). Philip Alan, Oxford.

Stewart, I. (1895) A uniform curriculum of education for nurses. *Nursing Record and Hospital World*, 2 November, 311–13, 9 November, 330–32, 16 November, 349–51, and 23 November, 370–2.

Stewart, I. (1898) 'The nursing conference, Miss Stewart's address'. *Nursing Record and Hospital World*, 25 June, 512.

Stewart, I. (1905) The twentieth century matron. *British Journal of Nursing*, 11 November, 392–6 and 18 November, 414–15.

Styles, M. (1985) 'Accountable to whom?' *International Nursing Review*, **32**, 73–5.

Sundram, C. (1986) 'Strategies to prevent patient abuse in public institutions'. *New England Journal of Human Services*, 6 (2), 20–5.

Symon, A. (2002) Midwifery Discipline: Misconduct and Negligence. Chapter 6. In: *Failure to progress: The contraction of the midwifery profession* (eds Mander, R. & Flaming, V.). Routledge, London.

Tew, M. (1995) *Safer childbirth? A critical history of maternity care.* Chapman & Hall, London.

Thompson, D. & Clare, J. (2002): http://www.dailytelegraph.co.uk/news/main.jhtml?xml=%2Fnews%2F2002%2F10%2F07%2Fnchas07.xml

Thompson, I.E., Melia, K.M. & Boyd, K.M. (1994) *Nursing Ethics*, 3rd edn. Churchill Livingstone, Edinburgh.

Thompson, T. (2001) Challenges and opportunities in education and training. In: *Community health care nursing* (eds Sines, D., Appleby, F. & Raymond, E.), 2nd edn. Blackwell Science, London.

Tierney, A.J., Taylor, J. & Closs, S.J. (1989) *A Study to Inform Nursing Support of Patients Coping with Chemotherapy for Breast Cancer.* Research Report, Nursing Research Unit, University of Edinburgh, Edinburgh.

Tierney, A.J. (1995) Accountability in nursing research. In: *Accountabilty in nursing* (ed. Watson, R.), pp. 209–31. Chapman & Hall, London.

Tierney, A.J., Closs, S.J., Hunter, H.C. & Macmillan, M.S. (1993) 'Experiences of elderly patients concerning discharge from hospital'. *Journal of Clinical Nursing*, **2**, 179–85.

Tilley, S. (1995) Accounts, accounting and accountability in psychiatric nursing. In: *Accountability in Nursing Practice* (ed. Watson, R.). Chapman & Hall, London.

Tilley, S. & Pollock, L. (1999) The two cultures of the Community Psychiatric Nurse: 'Twixt covenant and contract in work with "people with enduring mental disorders" '. Paper presented at the ICN conference, 29 June 1999, London.

Tilley, S. & Pollock, L. (2001) *'Prudent Empowerment, Sustaining Relationships: Themes in Community Psychiatric Nurses' Work with People with Enduring Mental Disorders.* Department of Nursing Studies, University of Edinburgh, Edinburgh.

Tingle, J.H. (1990) 'Ethics in practice'. *Nursing Times*, **86** (48), 54–5.

Tingle, J.H. (1991) 'Negligence: the new accountability'. *Nursing Standard*, 5 (29), 18–19.

Tingle, J. (2001a) Legal Aspects of Expanded Role. In: *Law and Nursing* (eds McHale, J. & Tingle, J.), 2nd edn, pp. 68–88. Butterworth Heinemann, Oxford.

Tingle, J. (2001b) Patient Complaints. In: *Law and Nursing* (eds McHale, J. & Tingle, J.), 2nd edn, pp. 48–67. Butterworth and Heinemann, Oxford.

Tingle, J. (2001c) Nursing Negligence: General Issues. In: *Law and Nursing* (eds McHale, J. & Tingle, J.), 2nd edn, pp. 26–47. Butterworth Heinemann, Oxford.

Tingle, J. (2002) Clinical Governance and the Law. In: *Clinical Governance: A Guide to Implementation for Healthcare Professionals* (eds McSherry, R. & Pearce, P.). pp. 115–25. Blackwell Science, Oxford.

Tingle, J. & Foster, C. (2002) *Clinical Guidelines: Law, Policy and Practice.* Cavendish Publishing, London.

Trainor, J., Pomeroy, E. & Pape, B. (1999) *Building a framework for support: a community development approach to mental health policy.* Canadian Association for Mental Health, Toronto.

Tschudin, V. (1989) *Ethics in Nursing: the caring relationship*, 1st edn. Heinemann Nursing, Oxford.

Tschudin, V. (1992) *Ethics in Nursing*, 2nd edn. Butterworth Heinemann, Oxford.

Turnbull, A. (2002) *The good and the bad and the gobbledegook: review of tackling NHS jargon.* Radcliffe Medical Press, Oxford.

Twinn, S. & Cowley, S. (1992) *The principles of health visiting: a re-examination.* Health Visitors' Association, London.

UKCC (1989) *Exercising Accountability.* United Kingdom Central Council for Nursing, Midwifery and Health Visiting, London.

UKCC (1992a) *Code of Professional Conduct*, 3rd edn. United Kingdom Central Council for Nursing, Midwifery and Health Visiting, London.

UKCC (1992b) *The Scope of Professional Practice.* United Kingdom Central Council for Nursing, Midwifery and Health Visiting, London.

UKCC (1996a) *Guidelines for Professional Practice.* United Kingdom Central Council for Nursing, Midwifery and Health Visiting, London.

UKCC (1996b) *Reporting Misconduct – information for employers and managers.* United Kingdom Central Council for Nursing, Midwifery and Health Visiting, London.

UKCC (1996c) *Reporting unfitness to practice – information for employers and managers. Issues arising from professional conduct complaints.* United Kingdom Central Council for Nursing, Midwifery and Health Visiting, London.

UKCC (1998a) *Guidelines for Mental Health and Learning Disabilities Nursing.* United Kingdom Central Council for Nursing, Midwifery and Health Visiting, London.

UKCC (1998b) *Complaints about Professional Conduct.* United Kingdom Central Council for Nursing, Midwifery and Health Visiting, London.

UKCC (1999a) *Practitioner-client relationships and the prevention of abuse.* United Kingdom Central Council for Nursing, Midwifery and Health Visiting, London.

UKCC (1999b) *Protecting the public – an employers guide to the United Kingdom Central Council for Nursing, Midwifery and Health Visiting registration confirmation service for nurses, midwives and health visitors.* United Kingdom Central Council for Nursing, Midwifery and Health Visiting, London.

UKCC (2001a) *Professional self-regulation and clinical governance. June 2001:* 3. United Kingdom Central Council for Nursing, Midwifery and Health Visiting, London.

UKCC (2001b) *Supporting Nurses, Midwives and Health Visitors through Lifelong Learning.* United Kingdom Central Council for Nursing, Midwifery and Health Visiting, London.

UKCC (2002) *Midwives rules and code of practice* (8 May 2002). United Kingdom Central Council for Nursing, Midwifery and Health Visiting, London: http://www.ukcc.org.uk/cms/content/publications/midwives.pdf (Accessed 18 July 2002).

United Nations Special Session on Children (2002): www.unicef.org/specialsession

Vaughan, B. (1989) 'Autonomy and accountability'. *Nursing Times,* 85 (3), 54–5.

Vehvilaeinen-Julkunen, K. (1993) 'The characteristics of clients and public health nurses in child health interactions'. *Scandinavian Journal of Caring Science,* 7, 11–16.

Walker, J. (1972) 'The changing role of the midwife'. *International Journal of Nursing Studies,* 9 (2), 85–94.

Walker, J. (1976) 'Midwife or obstetric nurse? Some perceptions of midwives and obstetricians of the role of the midwife'. *Journal of Advanced Nursing,* 1 (3), 129–38.

Walsh, M. (2000) *Nursing Frontiers: accountability & the boundaries of care.* Butterworth & Heinemann, Oxford.

Walsh, R. (2001) Autonomous roles in the community. In: *Community nursing and health care. Insights and innovations* (ed. Hyde, V.). Arnold, London.

Walshe, K. (1998a) 'Cutting to the heart of quality'. *Health Management,* 5, 20–1.

Walshe, K. (1998b) 'Clinical Governance; what does it really mean?' *Health Services Management Journal,* 4 (2), 1–2.

Walshe, K. (2000) *Clinical governance: a review of the evidence, November 2000.* Health Services Management Centre, University of Birmingham, Birmingham.

Walshe, K., Freeman, T., Latham, L., Wallace, L. & Spurgeon, P. (2000) *Clinical Governance: From Policy to Practice – Summary of Research Report.* The University of Birmingham, Birmingham.

Watson, R. (1992) 'Justifying your practice'. *Nursing,* 5 (3), 11–13.

Watson, R. (1995) *Accountability in nursing practice.* Chapman & Hall, London.

Watson, R. (2001) 'Restraint: its use and misuse in the care of older people'. *Nursing older people,* 13 (3), 21–5.

Watson, R. (2002) *Why do we have to learn this, we're only going to be nurses?* RCN Northern & Yorkshire & the Humber Research & Development Network – Grasping the Nettle: research activity in nursing, University of Bradford, Bradford.

Watson, R. & Manthorpe, J. (2002) 'Research Governance: for whose benefit?' *Journal of Advanced Nursing,* 39, 515–16.

Weinstein, J. (1998) The Professions and their inter-relationships. In: *Standards and Learning Disability* (eds Thompson, T. & Mathias, P.), 2nd edn. Balliere Tindall, London.

White, R. (1977) 'Accountability – a necessity for survival?' *Nursing Mirror*, 17 November, 25.

Wilensky, H. (1964) 'The Professionalisation of everyone?' *American Journal of Sociology*, 70, 137–58.

Williams, G. & Loder, C. (1990) The importance of quality and quality assurance. In: *Quality Assurance and Accountability in Higher Education* (ed. Loder, C.), pp. 1–12. University of London Institute of Higher Education, London.

Williams, S., Calnan, M., Cant, S.. & Coyle, J. (1993) 'All change in the NHS? Implications of the NHS reforms for primary care prevention'. *The Sociology of Health and Illness*, 15 (1), 43–67.

Williamson, O. (1975) *Markets and Hierarchies: Analysis and Antitrust Implications*. Free Press, New York.

Willis, J. (2001) *Friends in low places*. Radcliffe Medical Press, Oxford: www.friendsinlowplaces.co.uk

Wolfensberger, W. (1972) *The principal of normalisation in human management services*. National Institute of Mental Retardation, Toronto.

Wolverson, M. (2000) 'On reflection'. *Learning Disability Practice*, 3 (2), 24–7.

Wood, C. (1901) *A retrospect and a forecast*. Transactions of the Third International Congress of Nurses Pan-American Exposition, Buffalo, 18–21 September, p. 374.

Woodman, J. (1997) 'Nurse triage: easing the workload'. *Practice Nurse*, 14, 554–8.

World Health Organisation (1983) *The principles of quality assurance*. WHO, Copenhagen.

World Health Organisation (1986) *Charter for Health Promotion, WHO?* Canadian Public Health Alliance, Ottowa.

Zerwekh, J. (1992) The practice of empowerment and coercion by expert public health nurses. *Image: Journal of Nursing Scholarship*, 24 (2), 101–5.

Index